PRACTICAL ATLAS of
SKULL BASE
SURGERY

KOREAN SKULL BASE SOCIETY

PRACTICAL ATLAS OF
SKULL BASE SURGERY

1st Edition Printed | November 11, 2021
1st Edition Issued | November 27, 2021

Author	Korean Skull Base Society
Planned by	Andy Lim
Publisher	Ju-Yeon Chang
Edited by	Su-Jin Kim
Design by	Eun-Jung Yang
Cover Design by	Jae-Wook Kim
Illustrated by	Ho-Hyeon Lee
Publishing House	Koonja Publishing, Inc.

Registration No. 4-139 (June 24, 1991)
Paju Publishing Complex, 338, Hoedong-gil (474-1 Seopae-dong),
Paju-si, Gyeonggi-do, South Korea (10881)
Telephone: (031) 943-1888 Fax: (031) 955-9545
Website: www.koonja.co.kr

ISBN 979-11-5955-779-8

EDITORIAL BOARD

CONTRIBUTING AUTHORS

Hak Chang M.D., Ph.D.
Department of Plastic and Reconstructive Surgery, Seoul National University Hospital, Seoul, Republic of Korea

Ki-Hong Chang M.D., Ph.D.
Department of Otorhinolaryngology-HNS, Eunpyeong St. Mary's Hospital, Seoul, Republic of Korea

Kyung Gi Cho M.D., Ph.D.
Department of Neurosurgery, CHA Bundang Medical Center, Seongnam, Republic of Korea

Sung Jin Cho M.D., Ph.D.
Department of Neurosurgery, Soonchunhyang University Seoul Hospital, Seoul, Republic of Korea

Jong Woo Choi M.D., Ph.D.
Department of Plastic and Reconstructive Surgery, Asan Medical Center, Seoul, Republic of Korea

Sébastien Froelich M.D.
Department of Neurosurgery, Lariboisière Hospital, Paris, France

Bernard George M.D.
Department of Neurosurgery, Lariboisière Hospital, Paris, France

Chang-Ki Hong M.D., Ph.D.
Department of Neurosurgery, Asan Medical Center, Seoul, Republic of Korea

Je Beom Hong M.D.
Department of Neurosurgery, Kangbuk Samsung Hospital, Seoul, Republic of Korea

Jong Won Hong M.D., Ph.D.
Department of Plastic & Reconstructive Surgery, Severance Hospital, Seoul, Republic of Korea

Sang Duk Hong M.D., Ph.D.
Department of Otorhinolaryngology-HNS, Samsung Medical Center, Seoul, Republic of Korea

Beom Cho Jun M.D., Ph.D.
Department of Otorhinolaryngology-HNS, Uijeongbu St. Mary hospital, Gyeonggi, Republic of Korea

Shin Jung M.D., Ph.D.
Department of Neurosurgery, Chonnam National University Hwasun Hospital, Hwasun, Republic of Korea

Han Kyu Kim M.D., Ph.D.
Department of Neurosurgery, CHA Bundang Medical Center, Seongnam, Republic of Korea

Han Su Kim M.D., Ph.D.
Department of Otorhinolaryngology-HNS, Ewha womans university medical center, Seoul, Republic of Korea

Kyung Hwan Kim M.D., Ph.D.
Department of Neurosurgery, Chungnam National University Hospital, Daejeon, Republic of Korea

Yong Hwy Kim M.D., Ph.D.
Department of Neurosurgery, Seoul National University Hospital, Seoul, Republic of Korea

Young-Hoon Kim M.D., Ph.D.
Department of Neurosurgery, Asan Medical Center, Seoul, Republic of Korea

Doo-Sik Kong M.D., Ph.D.
Department of Neurosurgery, Samsung Medical
Center, Seoul, Republic of Korea

Kyu-Sung Lee M.D., Ph.D.
Department of Neurosurgery, Yonsei University
Health System, Seoul, Republic of Korea

Min Ho Lee M.D., Ph.D.
Department of Neurosurgery, Uijeongbu
St. Mary's Hospital, Gyeonggi, Republic of Korea

Seung Hwan Lee M.D., Ph.D.
Department of Neurosurgery, Kyung Hee University
Hospital at Gangdong, Seoul, Republic of Korea

Won Jae Lee M.D.
Department of Neurosurgery, Samsung Medical
Center, Seoul, Republic of Korea

Jaejoon Lim M.D., Ph.D.
Department of Neurosurgery, Bundang CHA
Medical Center, Seongnam, Republic of Korea

In Seok Moon M.D., Ph.D.
Department of Otorhinolaryngology, Gangnam
Severance Hospital, Seoul, Republic of Korea

Ju Hyung Moon M.D.
Department of Neurosurgery, Endoscopic Skull
Base Center, Severance Hospital, Seoul, Republic of Korea

Kyung-Sub Moon M.D., Ph.D.
Department of Neurosurgery, Chonnam National
University Hwasun Hospital . Jeollanam-do, Republic of
Korea

Sung-Il Nam M.D., Ph.D.
Department of Otorhinolaryngology-HNS, Dongsan
Hospital, Daegu, Republic of Korea.

Hyuk-Jin Oh M.D., Ph.D.
Department of Neurosurgery, SoonChunHyang
University Cheonan Hospital, Cheonan,
Republic of Korea

Tae Suk Oh M.D., Ph.D.
Department of Plastic and Reconstructive
Surgery, Asan Medical Center, Seoul,
Republic of Korea

Bong Jin Park M.D., Ph.D.
Department of Neurosurgery, Kyung Hee
Univerversity Medical Center, Seoul,
Republic of Korea

Ho Jin Park M.D., Ph.D.
Department of Plastic and Reconstructive
Surgery, Asan Medical Center, Seoul,
Republic of Korea

Hun Ho Park M.D., Ph.D.
Department of Neurosurgery, Gangnam
Severance Hospital, Seoul, Republic of Korea

Kwan Park M.D., Ph.D.
Department of neurosurgery, KonKuk University
Medical Center, Seoul, Republic of Korea

Ho Jun Seol M.D., Ph.D.
Department of Neurosurgery, Samsung Medical
Center, Seoul, Republic of Korea

FORWORD

Founded in 1994, the Korean Skull Base Society (KSBS) has a long-standing history of 28 years. Currently, about six hundred medical staff from various specialized fields such as neurosurgery, otolaryngology, plastic surgery and ophthalmology participate in research on surgical treatment of skull base disease. The Korean Skull Base Society is proud to be one of the most historical and multidisciplinary societies in Korea that investigates skull base disease.

Because of the complex nature of the skull base disease, the surgical process is highly complicated. It is even said to be one of the most challenging surgical fields where successful surgeries can only be achieved through the cooperation of several departments.

On behalf the Korean Skull Basel Society, I am beyond pleased to publish the first version of operative atlas in English. I hope that this book will be not only an educational guide for students majoring in the studies of the the skull base, but also a useful reference for those who actually operate in the professional surgical field.

I would like to express my gratitude to Editor-in-Chief Yong Hwy Kim and the editorial staff and writers who created this book in a short time with such enthusiasm and passion. I would also like to thank Koonja Publishing Company for bringing this book into the world.

I truly hope that this book will be helpful for those who perform operations in the field of skull base surgery.

Sung Jin Cho M.D., Ph.D.
President of Korean Skull Base Society
Department of Neurosurgery,
Soonchunhyang University Seoul Hospital,
Seoul, Republic of Korea

The solid and deep anatomical knowledge is the coner stones of skull base surgery. And the surgical techniques responding the diverse intraoperative situations are essential for the appliance and modification of standard approaches to optimize the exposure and resection of tumors and vascular lesions. And the reconstruction after skull base surgery the key steps for the safty and quality of life of patients.

The book's twenty-three chapters roughly divided into three sections, transcranial approaches, endoscopic approaches, and reconstructive surgeries. Each chapters dealt only the specifial skull base approaches for specific regions excluding the popular surgical techniques. Chapters begin with the brief introduction of surgical indication and relevant anatomic structures to help the quick overview of each surgical techniques. The main body was composed of the description of surgical techniques with the anatomical dissection and intraoperative photographs and illustration to improve the readers' understanding in the step-by-step fashion. The relevant anatomy encountered during the operation were also illustrated. The surgical tips and know-how were stressed in the text and figure legends and the key points of techniques were summarized at the end of chapters.

The goal of this book is to assist young neurosurgeon, otolaryngologists, head and neck surgeons and plastic surgeons to better understand the surgical anatomy. We hope that this volume will lead to improve the surgical techniques and bring the innovative idea for the better care of patients.

We could not imagine our knowledge and skills without the guidance and encouragement of our senior professors. Their spirit and passion have shaped who we are today. And All authors express our deep appreciation for the dedicated assistances from Andy Lim, Su Jin kim, Ho Hyeon Lee of Koonja Publisher to publish this book.

Personally, I would like to express my deep gratitude to my mentors, Hee Won Jung, Dong Gyu Kim and James J. Evans, who taught me to grow as a neurosurgeon.

Yong Hwy Kim M.D., Ph.D.
Editor-in-Chief
Department of Neurosurgery
College of Medicine, Seoul National University
Seoul National University Hospital

CONTENTS

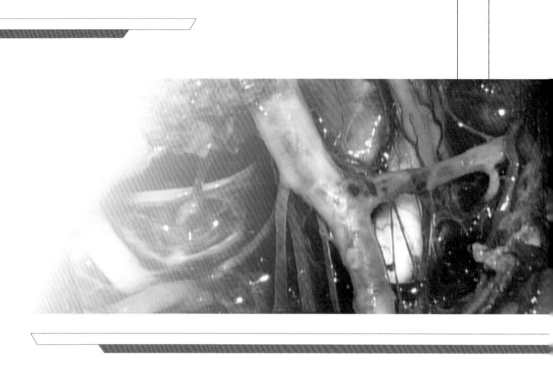

ORBITOZYGOMATIC APPROACH

Je Beom Hong M.D., Han Kyu Kim M.D., Ph.D.

I. Introduction

The orbitozygomatic approach can expand the space of access in the pterional approach by removing some of the superolateral rim of the orbit and zygoma. In the 1980s, Pellerin et al. and Hakuba et al. popular-ized this approach.[7,16]

This allows access to the subfrontal and subtempo-ral space while minimizing brain retraction, and also provides access to the parasellar area and interpedun-cular space.[6] Regions that can be accessed through the orbitozygomatic approach include orbital apex,

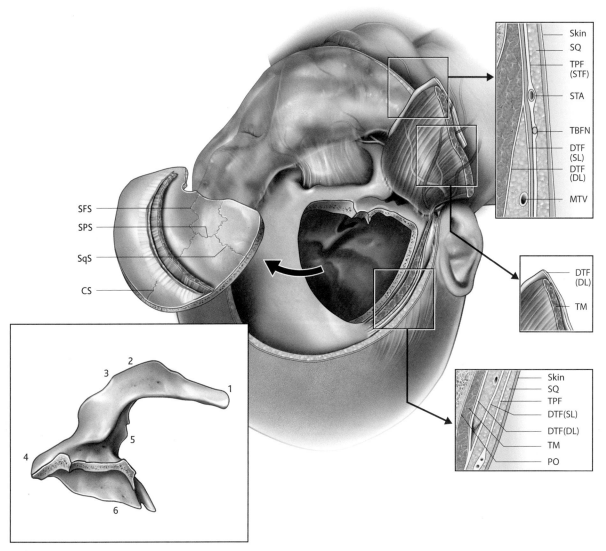

Figure 1-1. Overall illustration of the orbitozygomatic approach
DTF: deep temporal fascia, STA: superficial temporal artery, MTV: middle temporal vein, TM: temporalis muscle, SFAT: subcutaneous fibro-adipose tissue, STFP: superficial temporal fat pad, ZA: zygomatic arch, TPF: temporoparietal fascia, STF: superficial temporal fascia, GA: galea aponeurotica, LAT: loose areolar tissue, STFP: superficial temporal fat pad, SL: superficial layer, DL: deep layer, FZS: frontozygo-matic suture, SZS: sphenozygomatic suture, SFS: sphenofrontal suture, SPS: sphenoparietal suture, CS: coronal suture, SqS: squamous suture, IOF: inferior orbital fissure, SOF: superior orbital fissure, TBFN: temporal branch of facial nerve, number 1-6: orders of the bony cuts in orbitozygomatotomy.

paraclinoid regions, parasellar regions, cavernous sinus, interpeduncular regions, upper paraclival territories, and basilar apex. It can be used for surgery of pituitary macroadenomas, chordomas, sphenoid wing meningiomas, orbital meningiomas, petroclival meningiomas, trigeminal neurinomas, basilar tip aneurysms, anterior communicating artery aneurysms, and lesions of the cavernous sinus.

The orbitozygomatic approach is being carried out in several ways. The one-piece orbitozygomatic approach was introduced by Jane et al., and Al-Mefty et al.[1,9] The two-piece orbitozygomatic approach was introduced by Pellerin et al and Hakuba et al.[8,17,23] A 3-piece orbitozygomatic approach may be performed.[5] There are also various modified orbitozygomatic approaches.[2-4,6,12,14,20] In this article, the 2-piece orbitozygomatic approach will be described.

Anatomy to remember (Figure 1-1)

- MacCarty Keyhole can be made at the place about 5-6 mm back along the frontosphenoidal suture from the three suture junction (frontozygomatic suture, sphenofrontal suture, sphenozygomatic suture).[21] In other method, MacCarty keyhole is cut over the frontosphenoidal suture, about 1 cm behind the frontozygomatic junction.[20] Or it can be made at the place 7 mm above and 5 mm behind the sphenozygomatic suture to expose the periorbita and the frontal dura.[22] The MacCarty keyhole has an orbital roof in the middle, and the periorbita is exposed in the lower part and the frontal dura in the upper part.[15]
- Following the Sphenozygomatic suture can exposure the inferior orbital fissure (IOF).
- Following the frontozygomatic suture to the intraorbital perspective would lead to the superolateral portion of the superior orbital fissure (SOF).
- Zygomaticofacial foramen is the anteroinferior limit of osteotomy and becomes a landmark for cutting the zygoma. This is where the zygomaticofacial nerve from V2 passes. However there can be variations of the zygomaticofacial nerve and foramen.
- Transverse facial artery is a branch of STA and passes the lateral side of the zygomatic arch, so care should

be taken to avoid damage.
- Meningo-orbital band (MOB) is the frontotemporal dural fold in the superolateral side of SOF that is connected to the periorbita through the SOF. MOB is the medial limit of drilling, and when extradural anterior clinoidectomy is performed, it is cut.

II. Procedure

1. Position

1) Supine position, head elevation, shoulder elevation
2) Head rotated to the opposite side of the lesion about 30 degrees
3) Rotation can also be adjusted depending on the location of the lesion.
4) Neck extension (vertex down) allows the frontal lobe naturally to be separated from the orbital roof and helps to make the microsurgical view to the lesion from inferior to superior direction.

2. Skin incision

1) Curvilinear scalp incision
2) Start at 1 cm anterior to the tragus and extend to the contralateral mid-pupillary line just behind the hairline.
3) To preserve the temporal branch of the facial nerve, the skin incision should not cross under the zygomatic arch and do not exceed 2 cm anterior to the tragus.
4) Care must be taken to save the superficial temporal artery (STA) as well.

3. Dissection of scalp flap

1) Transareolar (subgaleal) dissection to elevate skin, subcutaneous tissue, and galea layers is performed.
2) Perform a dissection from the midline and proceed to the inferior until it meets the suprafascial fat pad.
3) Since the temporal branch of the facial nerve passes through the temporoparietal fascia, care must be taken to lift the superficial temporal fascia.[13,19] At this time, it can be performed in an interfascial fashion or a subfascial fashion.[12,18]
4) When using the interfascial dissection technique,

the superficial layer of the deep temporal fascia and the interfascial fat pad are lifted while dissection is performed over the deep layer of the deep temporal fascia to expose the zygoma.

5) When using the subfascial dissection technique, the superficial temporal fascia, fat pad, and deep temporal fascia are lifted all at once and dissection is performed to expose the zygoma. In this case, the zygoma surface can be exposed only when an incision is put in the deep layer of the deep temporal fascia on the medial side of the zygoma.

6) Interfascial-subperiosteal dissection or subfascial-subperiosteal dissection is performed to safely preserve the temporal branch of the facial nerve.

7) There is loose areolar tissue between the temporoparietal fascia (galea aponeurotica, superficial temporal fascia) layer and 2 layers of deep temporal fascia under it. There is a middle temporal vein and interfascial fat pad between these 2 layers.[10,11] (**Figure 2a, 2b**)

8) The zygomatic arch is below the deep layer of deep temporal fascia.

4. Temporalis muscle dissection

1) Leaving the musculofascial cuff along the superior temporal line can help with muscle reattachment during closure.

2) The retrograde dissection technique of the temporalis muscle and not using the monopolar cautery can help in preventing muscle atrophy and damaging nerves and blood vessels.

3) Be careful as the middle temporal artery and proximal medial branch of STA pass near the Zygomatic root.

4) After the temporalis muscle is detached, retraction in the inferior direction over the zygomatic arch exposes the middle cranial fossa.

5. Dissection of periorbita

1) Perform subperiosteal dissection to further expose the lateral orbital rim and zygoma. After that, the periorbita is dissected from the orbital wall and proceeds to the anterolateral portion of the IOF. Note that the superolateral aspect has a lacrimal

gland inside the lacrimal fossa.

2) Medial dissection can proceed to the supraorbital nerve that comes out through the supraorbital notch/foramen.

3) Care should be taken not to damage the periorbita during dissection from the zygomatic bone, orbital roof, superior and lateral wall of the orbit.

6. Craniotomy

1) In the 2-piece orbitozygomatic approach, standard pterional craniotomy is performed first, followed by orbitozygomatic bone flap.

2) MacCarty Keyhole can expose periorbita and frontal dura by making it about about 5-6 mm back along the frontosphenoidal suture from the three suture junction (frontzygomatic suture, sphenofrontal suture, sphenozygomatic suture) or MacCarty bur hole is cut over the frontosphenoidal suture, about 1 cm behind the frontozygomatic junction (**Figure 3a**).

3) orbitozygomatic craniotomy (**Figure 1-1, 3b**)

(1) It consists of a total of 6 cuts. The first is to do an oblique cut at the posterior root of the zygoma. At this time, it is performed right in front of the articular tubercle of the glenoid fossa to prevent damage to the temporomandibular joint.

(2) The second cut is done on the inferolateral margin of the zygoma above the zygomaticofacial foramen.

(3) The third cut starts at the anterolateral portion of the IOF and proceeds posterolaterally to meet the second cut on the malar eminence.

(4) The fourth cut starts vertically at the superior orbital rim and is performed on the orbital roof up to the SOF. The orbital roof is thin, so care must be taken not to damage the periorbita and prevent the periorbital fat coming out.

(5) The 5th cut starts at the IOF, the 6th cut starts at the SOF and connects the 3rd and 4th cuts.

(6) In closure, it is fixed using a miniplate and screw.

7. Drilling of basal structure

1) It is important to flatten the temporal base by drill-

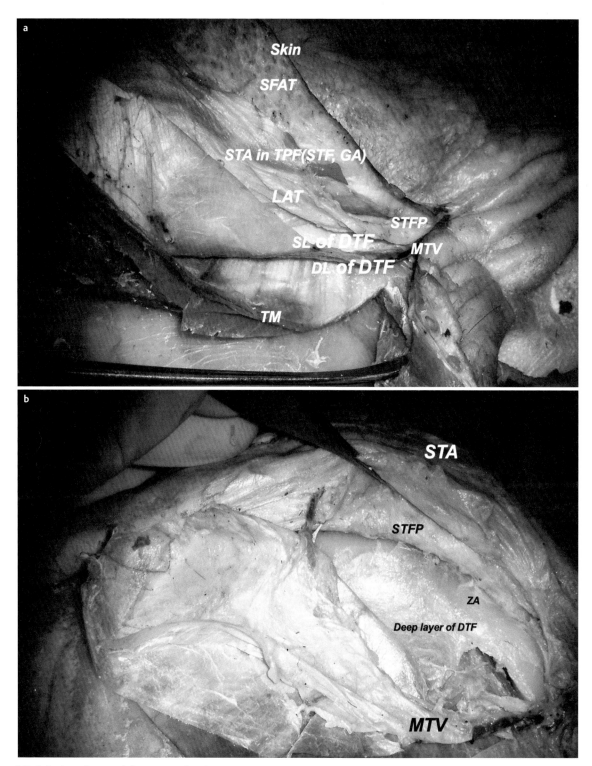

Figure 1-2. Soft tissue layers of the temporal region
DL: deep layer, DTF: deep temporal fascia, GA: galea aponeurotica, LAT: loose areolar tissue, MTV: middle temporal vein, SFAT: subcutaneous fibro-adipose tissue, STFP: superficial temporal fat pad, STA: superficial temporal artery, STF: superficial temporal fascia, STFP: superficial temporal fat pad, SL: superficial layer, TM: temporalis muscle, TPF: temporoparietal fascia, ZA: zygomatic arch

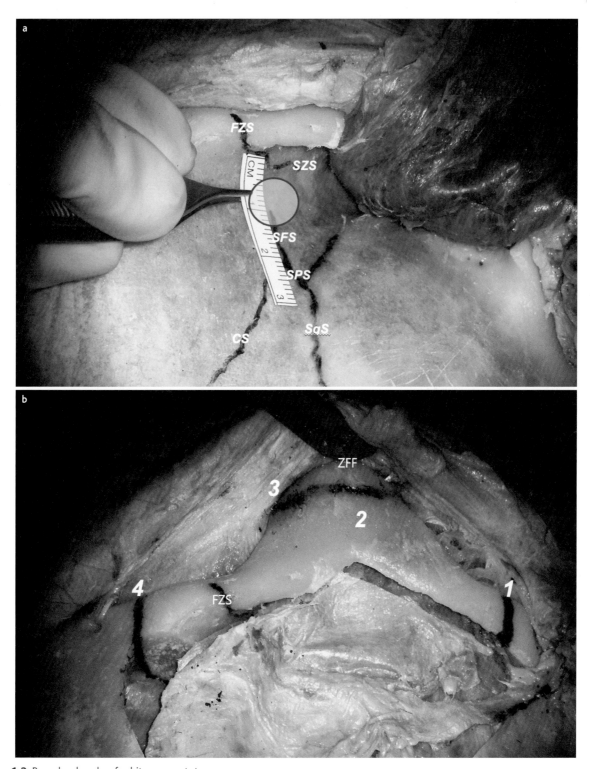

Figure 1-3. Bony landmarks of orbitozygomatotomy
FZS: frontozygomatic suture, SZS: sphenozygomatic suture, SFS: sphenofrontal suture, SPS: sphenoparietal suture, CS: coronal suture, SqS: squamous suture, ZFF: zygomaticofacial foramen
in Figure 3a, Yellow circle: position of MacCarty Keyhole, in Figure 3b, numbers indicate the order of zygomatic cuts.

ing the bones of the skull base when performing extradural anterior clinoidectomy, cavernous sinus approach, etc.

8. Dural opening

1) A dural incision is performed to include the lesion.

9. Closure

1) After intradural work, dura closure is made in a watertight fashion.
2) After that, the bone flap and zygoma are reapproximated and the temporalis muscle is sutured to its original position.

III. Illustrative case

A 55-year-old woman presented with general weakness, cognitive decline, dizziness, and visual disturbance. A clinoidal meningioma of about 8.4×8.3×8.2 cm size was found, and the tumor removal was planned to use an orbitozygomatic approach (**Figure 4a, 4b, 4c**).

The temporalis muscle was dissected in a subfascial-subperiosteal fashion to expose the superolateral rim and zygoma of the orbit (**Figure 5a**).

After extended pterional craniotomy, periorbita was dissected from the orbital rim (**Figure 5b**).

The anterolateral margin of the inferior orbital fissure was exposed (**Figure 5c**).

The periorbita was dissected from the lateral orbital rim to approach the inferior orbital fissure (**Figure 5d**).

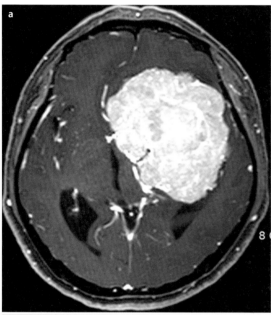

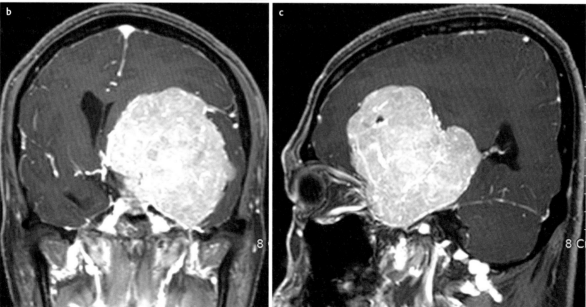

Figure 1-4. Illustrative case
T1 contrast enhanced axial (a), coronal (b), sagittal (c) magnetic resonance imaging (MRI).

Figure 1-5. Surgical steps of the illustrative case
(a) exposure of superficial temporal fat pad, superolateral wall of the orbital, zygomatic arch, frontozygomatic suture, FZS: frontozygomatic suture, STFP: superficial temporal fat pad
(b) periorbita dissection from superior orbital wall, PO: periorbita, FL: frontal lobe, TL: temporal lobe
(c) exposure of IOF, IOF: inferior orbital fissure
(d) periorbita dissection from lateral orbital wall to IOF
(e) orbitozygomatotomy bone flap

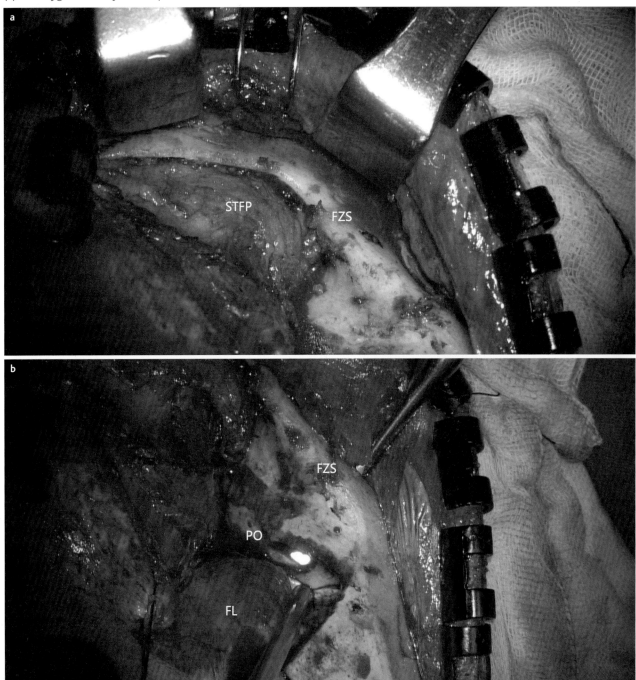

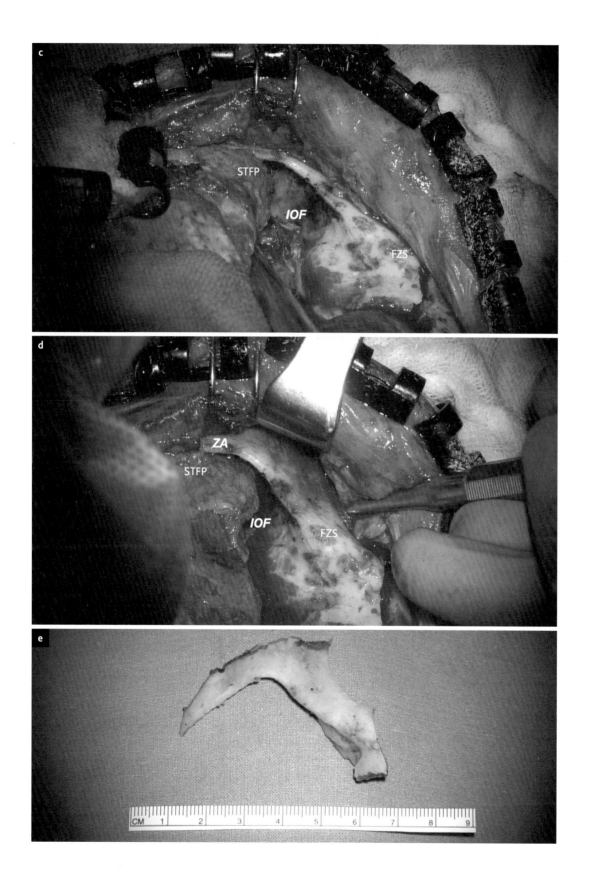

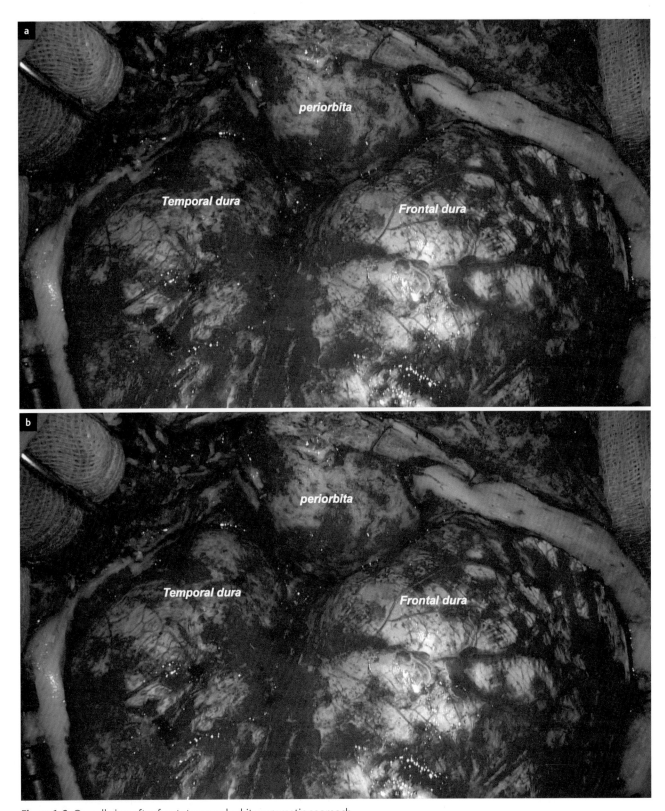

Figure 1-6. Overall view after frontotemporal orbitozygomatic approach

The orbitozygomatotomy was performed (**Figure 5e**).

Surgical view after orbitozygomatic osteotomy with extended pterional craniotomy (**Figure 6a, 6b**).

After that, an extradural anterior clinoidectomy was performed.

Opening the dura and removing the tumor will identify the ICA, A1, M1, and extradural optic nerves (**Figure 7a, 7b**).

After the tumor has been removed, we identified the neurovascular structures that can be exposed via

Figure 1-7. Intraoperative findings
(a) tumor dissection from vessels, ICA: internal carotid artery
(b) tumor dissection from ICA, optic nerve (CN II)
(c) final view after tumor removal, II: optic nerve, III; oculomotor nerve, SCA: superior cerebellar artery, PCoA: posterior communicating artery, AChoA: anterior choroidal artery

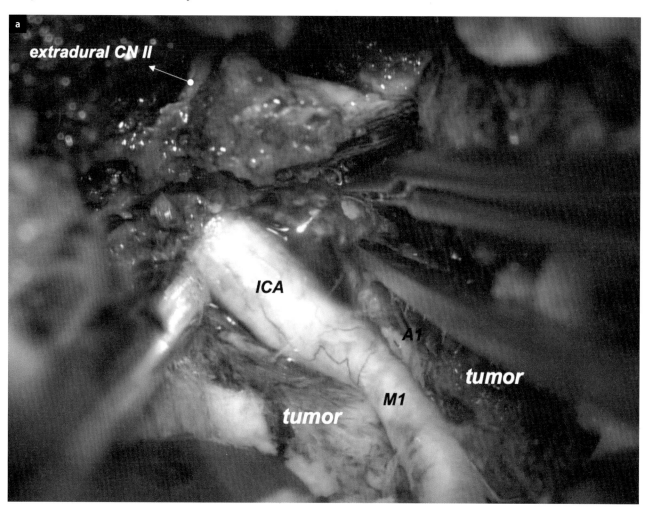

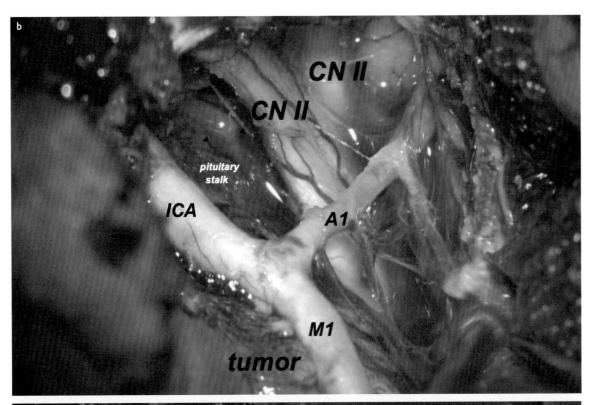

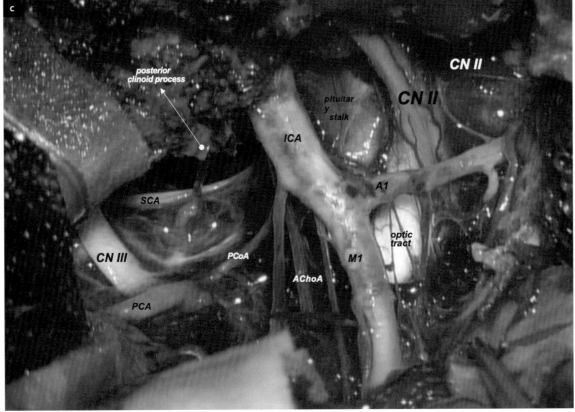

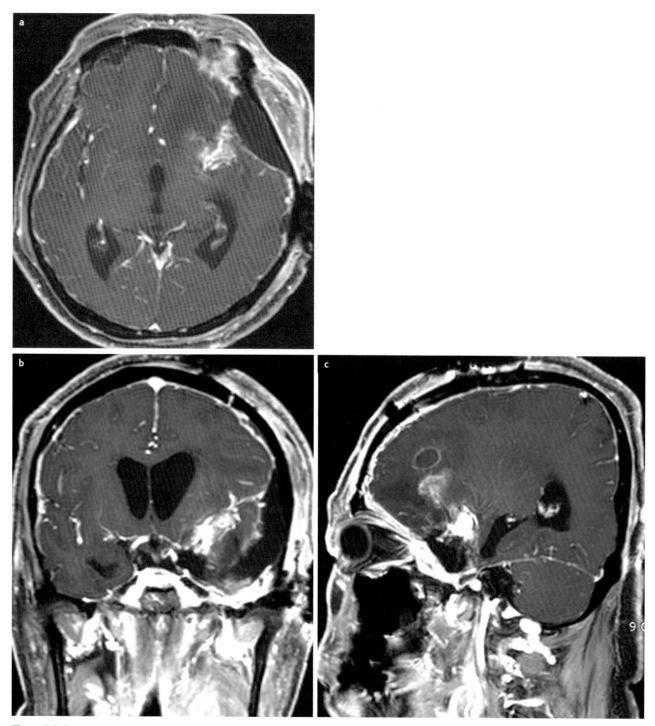

Figure 1-8. Postoperative MRI
T1 contrast enhanced axial (a), coronal (b), sagittal (c) MRI.

the orbitozygomatic approach (**Figure 7c**).

MRI performed after surgery can confirm that the tumor has been sufficiently removed (**Figure 8**).

IV. Surgical tip & pitfall

- Make a MacCarty keyhole to secure periorbita and frontal dura.
- Temporal branch of facial nerve passes through temporoparietal fascia (superficial temporal fascia, galea aponeurotica) or superficially, so dissection of the temporal fascia should be performed in interfascial dissection fashion or subfascial dissection fashion to expose zygoma and orbit.
- Frontotemporal branch of the facial nerve that courses within the interfascial space and then enters the frontalis muscle in 30%.[20] Keep in mind that there may be damage to the facial nerve in the interfascial space.
- When dissecting the periorbita from the orbital rim, thin orbital roof or thin periorbita may be damaged. So care should be taken not to damage the periorbita.
- To prevent atrophy of temporalis muscle, the dissection can be performed in a subperiosteal retrograde fashion, saving STA and avoiding monopolar coagulation.
- Since there may be hyperostosis of the orbital roof in meningioma surgery, indiscriminate and blind fracture of the orbital roof may cause damage to the optic canal and optic nerve and should be avoided.[6]

REFERENCES

1. Al-Mefty O. Supraorbital-pterional approach to skull base lesions. Neurosurgery 1987;21(4):474-7.

2. Andaluz N, van Loveren HR, Keller JT, Zuccarello M. Anatomic and clinical study of the orbitopterional approach to anterior communicating artery aneurysms. Neurosurgery 2003;52(5):1140-9.

3. Balasingam V, Noguchi A, McMenomey SO, Delashaw JB Jr. Modified osteoplastic orbitozygomatic craniotomy. Technical note: Technical note. J Neurosurg 2005;102(5):940-4.

4. Bilbao CJ, Stofko DL, Dehdashti AR. Cranio-orbitozygomatic approach: Technique and modifications. Oper Tech Otolayngol Head Neck Surg 2013;24(4):229-34.

5. Campero A, Martins C, Socolovsky M, Torino R, Yasuda A, Domitrovic L, et al. Three-piece orbitozygomatic approach. Neurosurgery 2010;66 (3 Suppl Operative):E119-20; discussion E120.

6. Cohen-Gadol A. The orbitozygomatic craniotomy and its judicious use. Oper Neurosurg (Hagerstown) 2020;18(5):559-69.

7. Hakuba A, Liu S, Nishimura S. The orbitozygomatic infratemporal approach: a new surgical technique. Surg Neurol 1986;26(3):271-6.

8. Hakuba A, Liu Ss, Shuro N. The orbitozygomatic infratemporal approach: A new surgical technique. Surgical Neurology 1986;26:271-6.

9. Jane JA, Park TS, Pobereskin LH, Winn RH, Butler AB. The supraorbital approach: Technical note. Neurosurgery 1982;11(4):537-42.

10. Jung W, Youn K-H, Won S-Y, Park J-T, Hu K-S, Kim H-J. Clinical implications of the middle temporal vein with regard to temporal fossa augmentation. Dermatol Surg 2014;40(6):618-23.

11. Kapoor KM, Bertossi D, Li CQ, Saputra DI, Heydenrych I, Yavuzer R. A systematic literature review of the middle temporal vein anatomy: "venous danger zone" in temporal Fossa for filler injections. Aesthetic Plast Surg 2020;44(5):1803-

12. Kodera T, Arishima H, Yamada S, Arai H, Akazawa A, Higashino Y, et al. Orbitozygomatic craniotomy with modified Zabramski's technique: A technical note and anatomic and clinical findings. World Neurosurg 2017;97:49-57.

13. Krayenbühl N, Isolan GR, Hafez A, Yaşargil MG. The relationship of the fronto-temporal branches of the facial nerve to the fascias of the temporal region: a literature review applied to practical anatomical dissection. Neurosurg Rev 2007;30(1):8-15.

14. Lemole GM Jr, Henn JS, Zabramski JM, Spetzler RF. Modifications to the orbitozygomatic approach. Technical note: Technical note. J Neurosurg 2003;99(5):924-30.

15. MacCarty CS. The surgical treatment of intracranial meningiomas. The Surgical Treatment of Intracranial Meningiomas 1961.pp.57-60.

16. Pellerin P, Lesoin F, Dhellemmes P, Donazzan M, Jomin M. Usefulness of the orbitofrontomalar approach associated with bone reconstruction for frontotemporosphenoid meningiomas. Neurosurgery 1984;15(5):715-8.

17. Rodriguez Rubio R, Chae R, Kournoutas I, Abla A, McDermott M. Immersive surgical anatomy of the frontotemporal-orbitozygomatic approach. Cureus 2019;11(11):e6053.

18. Salas E, Ziyal IM, Bejjani GK, Sekhar LN. Anatomy of the frontotemporal branch of the facial nerve and indications for interfascial dissection. Neurosurgery 1998;43(3):563-8; discussion 568-9.

19. Seçkin H, Avci E, Uluç K, Niemann D, Başkaya MK. The work horse of skull base surgery: orbitozygomatic approach. Technique, modifications, and applications. Neurosurg Focus 2008;25(6):E4.

20. Shimizu S, Tanriover N, Rhoton AL Jr, Yoshioka N, Fujii K. MacCarty keyhole and inferior orbital fissure in orbitozygomatic craniotomy. Neurosurgery 2005;57(1 Suppl):152-9; discussion 152-9.

21. Tubbs RS, Loukas M, Shoja MM, Cohen-Gadol AA. Refined and simplified surgical landmarks for the MacCarty keyhole and orbitozygomatic craniotomy. Neurosurgery 2010;66(6 Suppl Operative): 230-3.

22. Zabramski JM, Kiriş T, Sankhla SK, Cabiol J, Spetzler RF. Orbitozygomatic craniotomy. Technical note: Technical note. J Neurosurg 1998;89(2):336-41.

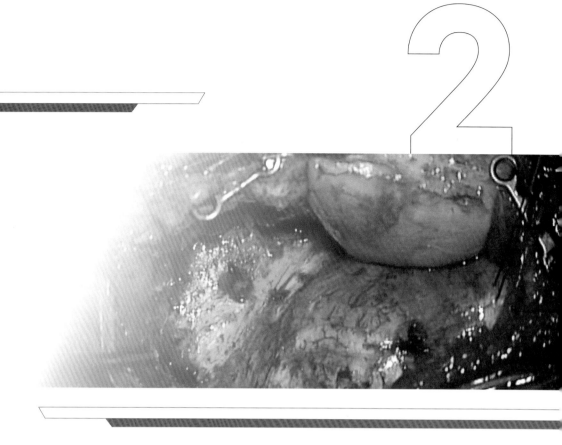

MODIFIED LATERAL SUPRA-ORBITAL (MLSO) APPROACH

Jaejoon Lim M.D., Ph.D., Kyung Gi Cho M.D., Ph.D.

I. Introduction

The pterional approach is one of the basic approaches for anterior skull lesions. The orbitozygomatic approach is selected when expansion of the corridors in the realm of anterior cranial fossa is needed. To enhance the completeness and cosmetics following surgery, several approaches have been developed and modified based on the pterional approach. Among them, Modified Lateral Supra-Orbital (MLSO) approach could be one of the best approaches, which was devised to obtain the merit of pteriornal, orbitozygomatic, lateral supraorbital and supraorbital keyhole approaches. Generally, this approach could be used for accessing the lesions in the frontal lobe, orbit, olfactory groove, suprasellar and parasellar area, sphenoid ridge, cavernous sinus, frontotemporal area. Some lesions of the upper clivus, anterior petroclival junction and cerebellopontine angle may be accessed by this approach.

II. Procedure

1. Position

The patient is positioned in a supine position with the head fixed by the head holder. The head is elevated above the heart and turned toward the contralateral side by 10° to 45° depending on the lesion location. Also, the degree of head extension is determined by location of the lesion. When the lesion is in the middle of the anterior frontal base, optimal rotational angle would be between 30° to 45°. In case the lesion is in the frontotemporal or posterior area, 10° to 30° head rotation would be adequate. Additional head extension would be needed for lesions in the suprasellar or 3rd ventricle area (**Figure 2-1**).

2. Skin incision

The skin incision is located at the inferior edge of the eyebrow, starting from 0.5 cm medial to the mid-pupillary line. The skin incision could be extending laterally to just behind the frontal process of the zygomatic bone and approximately 1 cm inferior laterally (**Figure 2-2**).

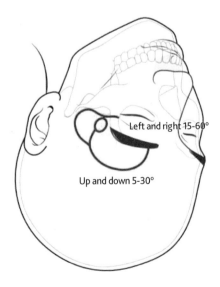

Left and right 15-60°

Up and down 5-30°

Figure 2-1. Position of MLSO

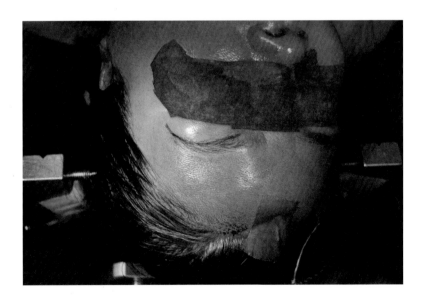

3. Craniotomy and bone flap

To expose the frontal bone and temporalis fascia, subcutaneous dissection was performed carefully, so as not to damage the supraorbital nerve. After making an incision of about 2 cm in the temporal fascia, the temporal muscle was detached from the temporal bone to expose the pterion. Then, the temporal muscle was retracted with privately designed muscle hooks (**Figure 2-3, 4, 5**).

1) Cut the zygoma arch and the frontal bone with thin craniotome
2) A burr hole is drilled on the frontosphenoid suture
3) Fracture the orbital roof and the lateral orbital wall an osteotome
4) Free bone flap was made with a craniotome, including the supraorbital bone, frontozygomatic process and frontal bone.
5) The temporal bone is removed using a rongeur and punch. The temporal dura is exposed enough.

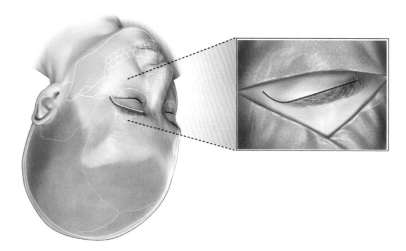

Figure 2-2. Skin incision of MLSO

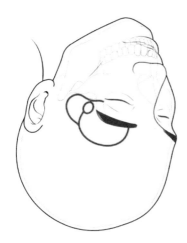

Figure 2-3. Craniotomy

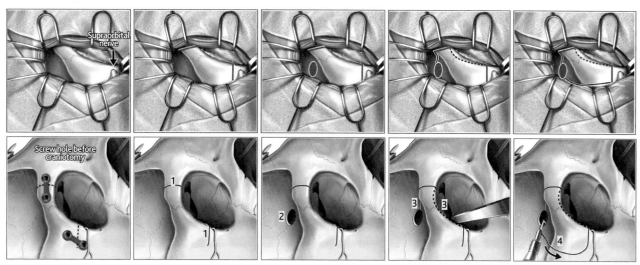

Figure 2-4. Craniotomy part I

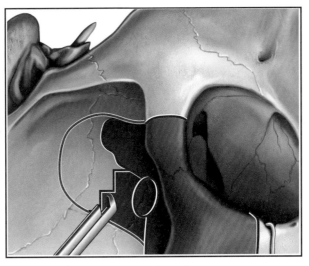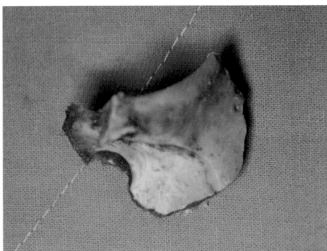

Figure 2-5. Craniotomy Part II and bone flap

4. Extradural anterior clinoidectomy

Extradural anterior clinoidectomy can be performed without difficulty after stepwise drilling of the orbital roof, lesser sphenoid wing, and optic strut. (See chapter 3 for detailed technique of anterior clinoidectomy) **(Figure 2-6)**

5. Anterior petrosectomy

The outer layer of the cavernous sinus is peeled extradurally from anterior to posterior, exposing the inner membranous layer. The greater superficial petrosal nerve is the lateral landmark, the anteromedial margin of the eminencia arcuata is the posterior landmark, and the lateral margin of the porus trigeminus

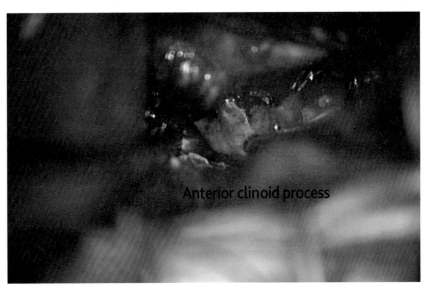

Figure 2-6. Extradual anterior clinoidectomy

is the posterior landmark in the middle cranial fossa. After confirming the anatomical landmarks of the Kawase triangle, the apex of the petrous bone is drilled out (**Figure 2-7**).

6. Frontal and temporal dura exposure

Frontal and temporal dura are fully exposed and extradural surgical field is enough to operation (**Figure 2-8**).

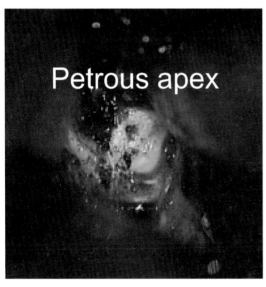

Figure 2-7.

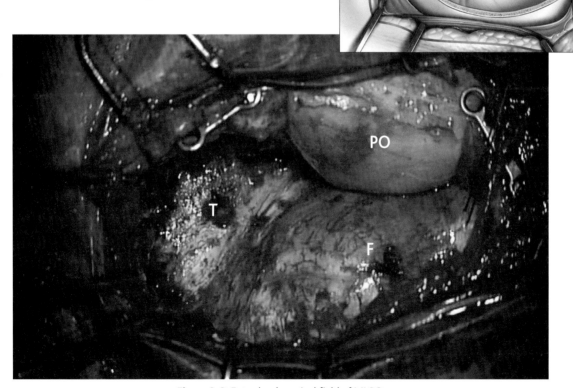

Figure 2-8. Extradural surgical field of MLSO.

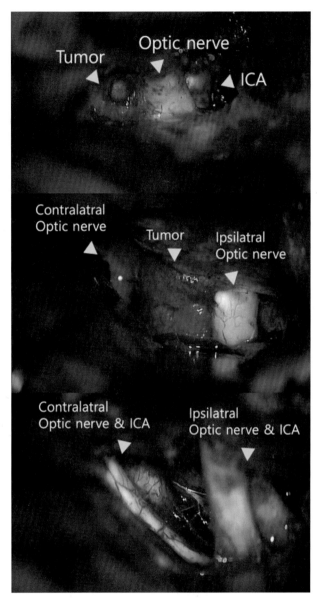

Figure 2-9. Intradural surgical field of MLSO.

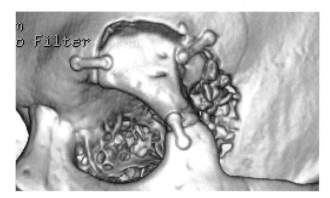

Figure 2-10.

7. Surgical picture of MLSO

The path of the optic nerve could be easily identified. It was possible to easily reach the medial area of the contralateral optic nerve through MLSO. The closed and direct view of the anterior frontal base lesion was possible through MLSO. It is possible to access the contralateral anterior skull base lesion as well as the ipsilateral through MLSO (Figure 2-9).

8. Bone flap fixation and closure

A mini cranial plate is used to fix the bone flap and a bone chip is used to fill the temporal craniectomy site. Careful skin wound closure is required to avoid cosmetic problem (Figure 2-10).

III. Clinical case of tuberculum sellae meningioma through MLSO approach

The preoperative diagnosis was tuberculum sellae meningioma. The MLSO approach was selected because the tumor removal and tumor origin dura manipulation were considered possible. A lower eyebrow incision was performed. The craniotomy was done including frontal and temporal bone. After MOB was cut, the anterior clinoidectomy was performed easily and completely. The tumor was directly identified via a dura incision from the frontal dura to the temporal dura. The gross total removal of the tumor was performed, then the tumor origin dura was removed. The Simpson Grade II resection was achieved. The postoperative Magnetic resonance imaging (MRI) showed the complete removal of the tumor. The pathological diagnosis was meningothelial meningioma (WHO grade I). The patient recovered without any complication (Figure 2-11).

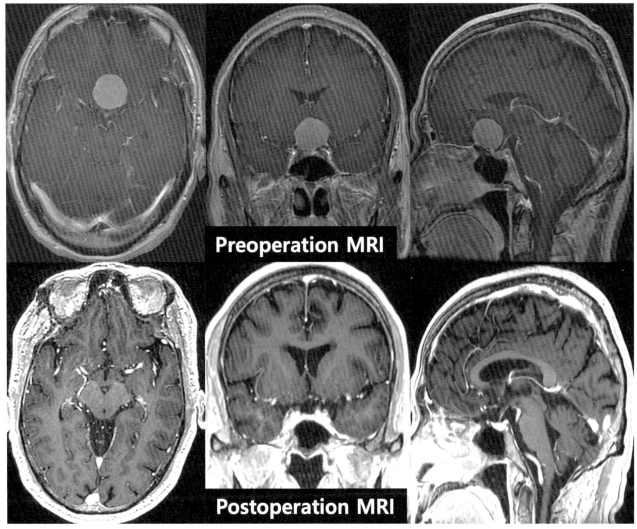

Figure 2-11. Preoperation and postoperation MRI of Tubercullum sellae meningioma

IV. Tip & Summary

1. The craniectomy site is relatively small compared to conventional pterional and orbitozygomtic approach.

   It takes time for being familiar with MLSO approach.

2. Enough temporal bone removal is important to secure surgical space.

3. Long surgical instruments can help to posterior fossa surgery.

4. Retraction of the periorbita can help to secure surgical space.

5. Be careful to avoid frontal sinus and ethmoid sinus infection.

6. In case of large-size tumor and severe brain edema, the MLSO approach may not be an appropriate.

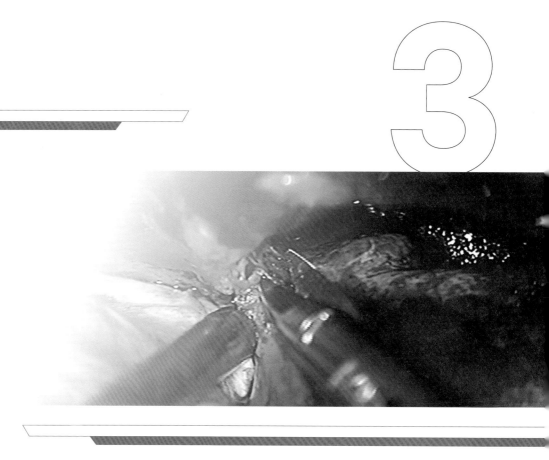

3

ANTERIOR CLINOIDECTOMY

Seung Hwan Lee M.D., Ph.D., Bong Jin Park M.D., Ph.D.

I. Introduction

The anterior clinoid process (ACP) is a portion of the posterior edge of the lesser wing of sphenoid bone projecting medially and posteriorly having a triangle shape. Two major bridges support this structure, one of which is a thin bone located anteriorly and medially, forming the roof of the optic canal, finally ending with planum sphenoidale. And the other is an optic strut that forms the lateral and inferior wall of the optic canal and separates it from the superior orbital fissure. The major structures around the ACP are as follows.

1) Optic nerve: ACP forms the lateral wall of the optic canal where the optic nerve passes from the posteromedial to the anterolateral direction.
2) Internal carotid artery (ICA): ICA lies underneath the ACP medioinferiorly, of which segment corresponds to the ophthalmic segment (C6).

3) Nerves within the superior orbital fissure: lacrimal, oculomotor, trochlear, ophthalmic (V1), and abducens nerves (listed from medial to lateral) pass via superior orbital fissure.

Anterior clinoidectomy is required to enhance maneuverability of the optic nerve and ICA in which pathologies reside near them. Representative techniques are divided into intradural and extradural clinoidectomy. The pros and cons of each technique are summarized below (**Table 3-1**).

1. Indication

Provided that opticocarotid and caroticooculomotor windows could be enlarged by the anterior clinoidectomy, stresses on the optic nerve and ICA either by pathology itself or manipulations during the surgery are to be reduced. Following pathologies can be more advantageous when anterior clinoidectomy is performed before the main procedure (**Table 3-2**).

Table 3-1. Comparison of characteristics between intradural and extradural clinoidectomy.

	Advantage	Disadvantage
Intradural	• It can provide direct visual confirmation of the important intradural neurovascular structures. • Enables tailored clinoidectomy according to the pathology. • Useful with ACP variation including coexistence of caroticoclinoid foramen and interosseous bridge.	• Can injure the critical structures by drilling. • Drilling by-products accumulate in the subarachnoid space. • CSF leakages often occur when ACP is pneumatized. • Unable to perform when the pathology resides on the ACP such as clinoidal meningioma.
Extradural	• It can have dural protection for the adjacent neurovascular structures. • Allows earlier devascularization of the tumor • Drilling by-products such as bone dust can be prevented. • Fewer cerebrospinal fluid leakage in case that ACPs are pneumatized as long as the integrity of the dura maintain • Provides the increased maneuverability at the beginning of the dissection in case of tumor pathology.	• Requires peeling the dura propria off the lateral wall of the cavernous sinus. • Suboptimal visual confirmation of adjacent neurovascular structure

Table 3-2. Pathologic lesions which can be helpful when anterior clinoidectomy is performed prior to main prodecure.

Vascular lesions	• Aneurysms on paraophthalmic ICA or basilar bifurcation.

Tumors	• Meningiomas around the ACP and optic nerve
	  - Clinoidal
	  - Medial sphenoid wing
	  - Cavernous sinus
	  - Tuberculum sellae
	• Craniopharyngioma
	• Pituitary adenoma

2. Preoperative preparation

1) Thin sliced CT in all 3 planes (axial, sagittal, coronal section)
   - To identify the shape of ACP and its composition whether to have pneumatization or not.
   - To estimate the angle orientation of the optic strut
2) Thin-sliced MR (T1, T1(e), and T2 sequences) for grasping eloquent structures around the lesion (transformed optic nerve and ICA)

II. Illustrative Case.

1. Presentation and image findings

A 49-year-old female patient was admitted for a headache and nausea that began a week ago. A brain computed tomography (CT) taken as an initial brain imaging study disclosed a mass that shows slight high density on plain CT and a relatively well-enhanced mass above the right clinoid process (**Figure 3-1**). Further, a sellar magnetic resonance (MR) imaging with gadolinium enhancement demonstrated a mass based on the right clinoid process showing homogenous enhancement. The measured sizes are 32×31×28 mm (width, length, and height) and severe displacement of right optic nerve toward medial direction is observed on T2-weighted image sequence (**Figure 3-2**). However, her right vision has not been considerably deteriorated, only showing limited rim defect on the visual field test (**Figure 3-3**). To prevent worsening of her vision, elective surgery for the removal of the clinoidal meningioma was indicated with extradural anterior clinoidectomy to aid early mobilization of the right optic nerve.

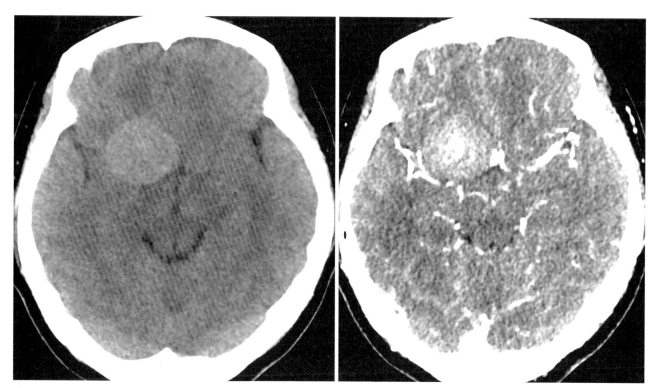

Figure 3-1. Computed tomography taken in the emergency department before admission discloses an oval hyperdense lesion at the right orbitofrontal lobe.

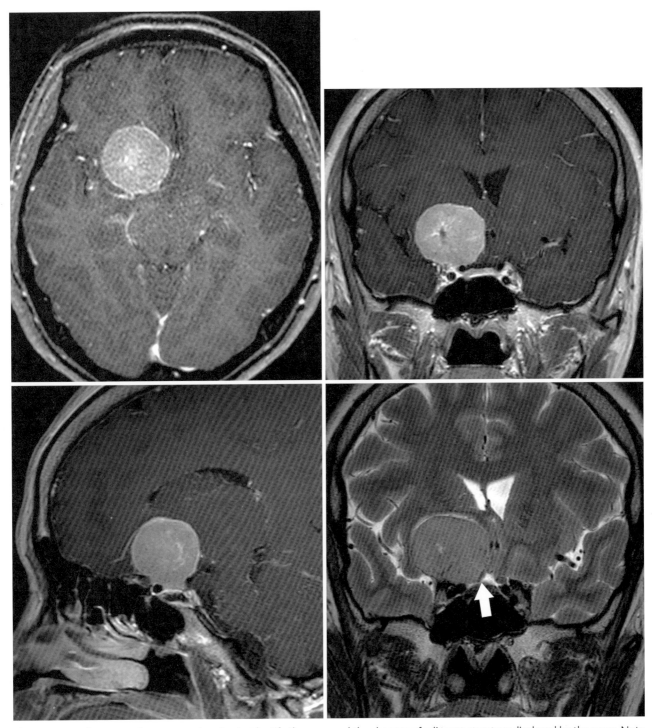

Figure 3-2. A sellar magnetic resonance imaging to identify the mass and the changes of adjacent structure displaced by the mass. Note that the left optic nerve is severely compressed and shifted medially (arrow).

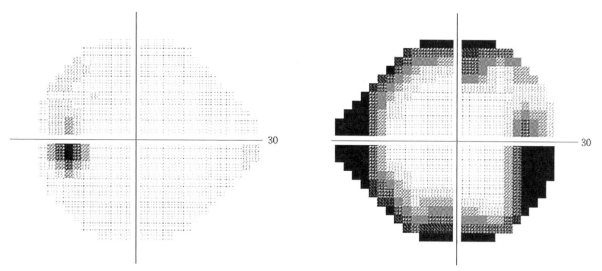

Figure 3-3. Pre-operative visual field test. There shows a 360-degree rim-shaped visual defect in the patient's right vision.

2. Surgical procedure

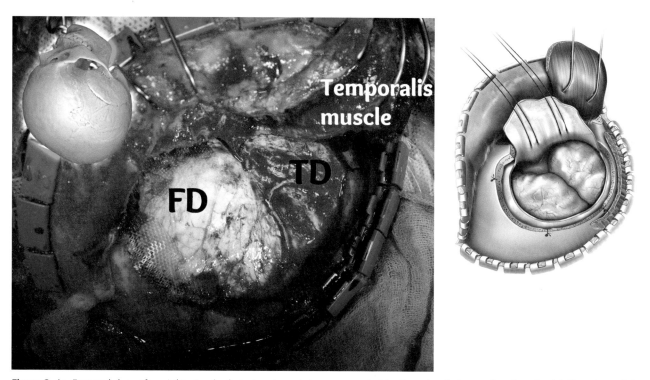

Figure 3-4a. Exposed dura after right standard pterional craniotomy, preceded by three burrhole creation, interfascial dissection of the temporalis muscle, and C-shaped skin incision made from posterior to the hairline to the zygomatic process. To help understanding the orientation of the head, a skull model is placed on the left upper portion of the figure.
FD, frontal dura; TD, temporal dura

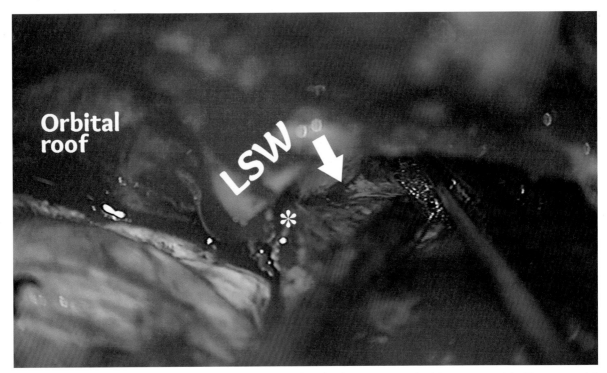

Figure 3-4b. Detaching the frontal dura from and drilling the orbital roof is the 1st step to obtain space to work in. The temporal dura is to be peeled away toward the posterior and medial direction until meningo-orbital band(*) is exposed. The meningo-orbital band is located at the most lateral portion of the superior orbital fissure.
Arrow indicates dural cuff enfolding into the superior orbital fissure. LSW, lesser sphenoid wing; asterisk, meningo-orbital band

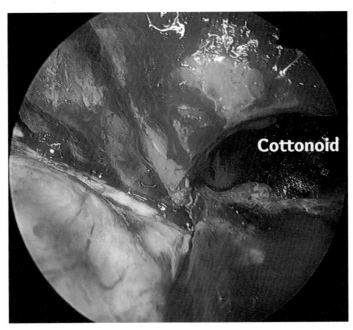

Figure 3-4c. Endoscopic view at the same stage of figure 3-4b to provide better visualization of deeper temporal area (greater wing of sphenoid bone). Hemostatic material and cottonoid are packed at the temporal base to control venous bleeding.

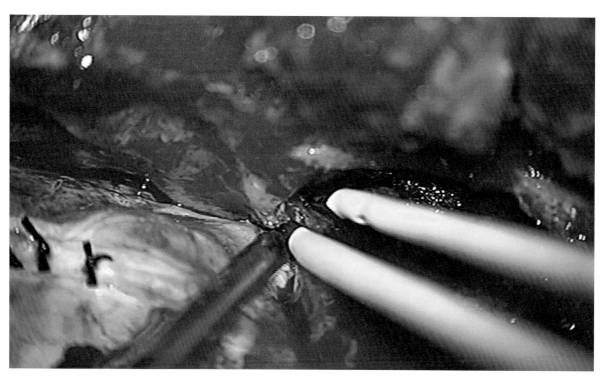

Figure 3-4d. Coagulation of the meningo-orbital band containing meningo-orbital artery is essential before the transaction.

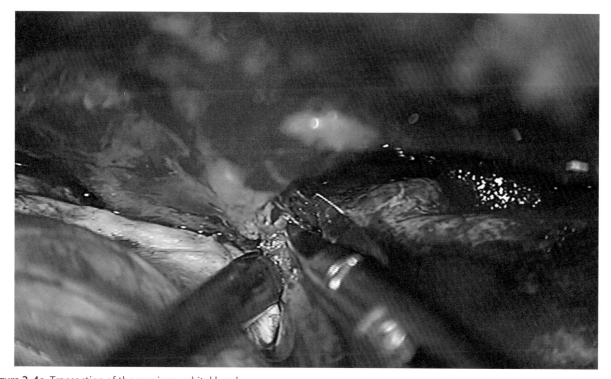

Figure 3-4e. Transaction of the meningo-orbital band.

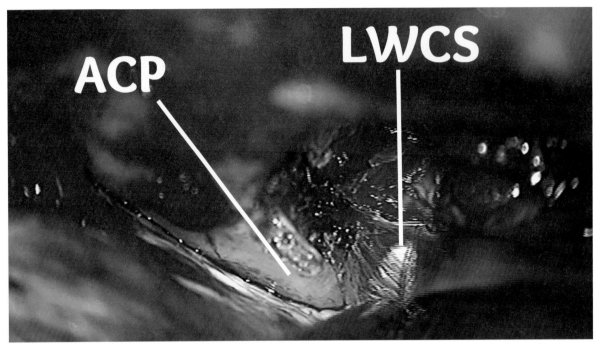

Figure 3-4f. A peeling of temporal dura from the lateral wall of the cavernous sinus allows the anterior clinoid process to be exposed, which eases the following drilling by providing sufficient space.
ACP, anterior clinoid process; LWCS, lateral wall of the cavernous sinus.

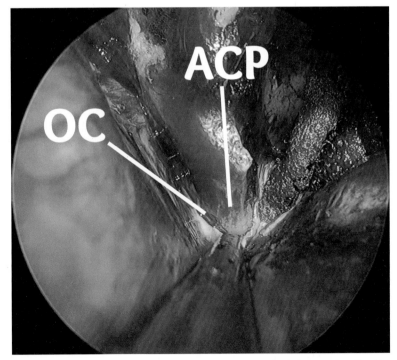

Figure 3-4g. Endoscopic inspection at the same step of figure 3-4f. The whole length of the anterior clinoid process (ACP), as well as the optic canal (OC), can be seen.

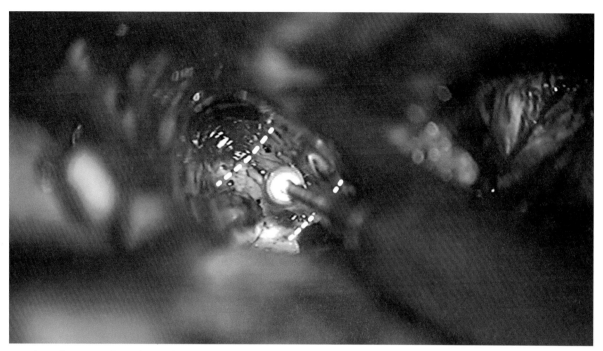

Figure 3-4h. Drilling starts from the medial edge of the optic canal toward the lateral side with a 2 mm diamond ball to unroof the optic canal. To protect the optic nerve from thermal injury, continuous saline cooling irrigation should be carried out. The passage of the right optic nerve is seen as dotted lines.

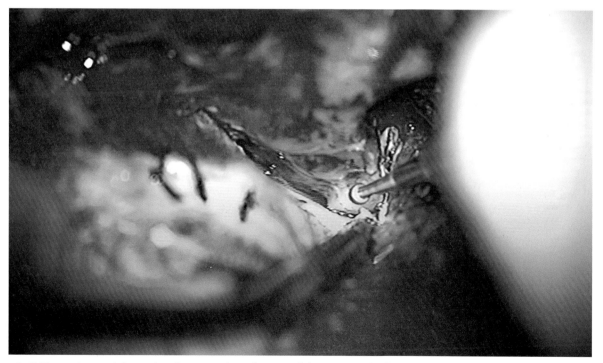

Figure 3-4i. The optic strut is located at the posterolateral corner of the optic canal, which needs to be drilled to disconnect the anterior clinoid process both from the roof of the optic canal and the lesser sphenoid wing.

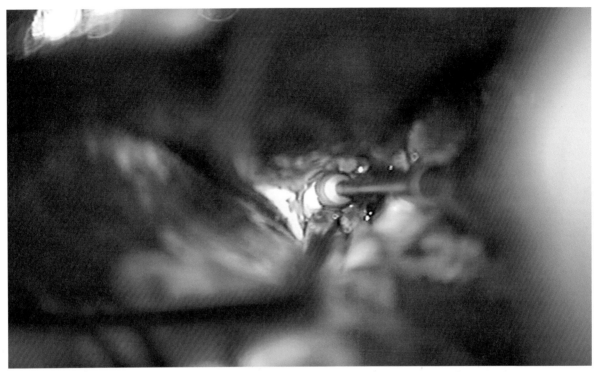

Figure 3-4j. For safety, the anterior clinoid process must be hollowed out with the diamond drill until a thin eggshell-like bone chip remains.

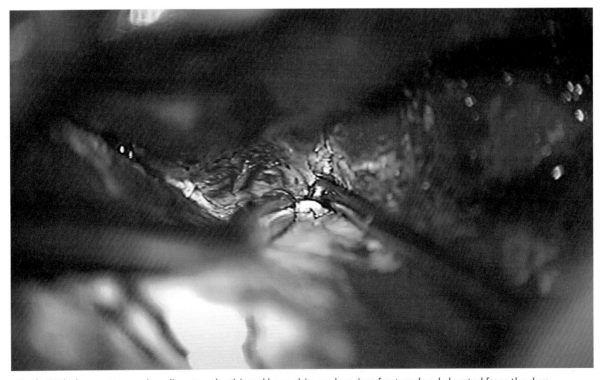

Figure 3-4k. With the curette or micro dissector, the thinned bone chip can be micro fractured and elevated from the dura.

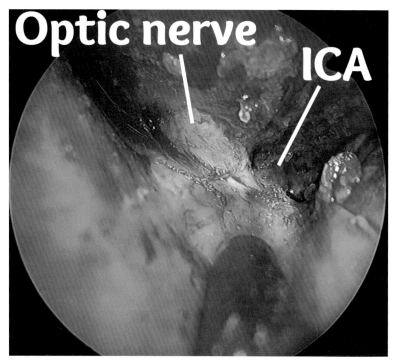

Figure 3-4l. An endoscopic photograph was taken after removal of the anterior clinoid process. The clinoid segment of the internal carotid artery is exposed, which lies between the proximal and distal dural ring. Unroofed optic nerve within the dura also is seen.

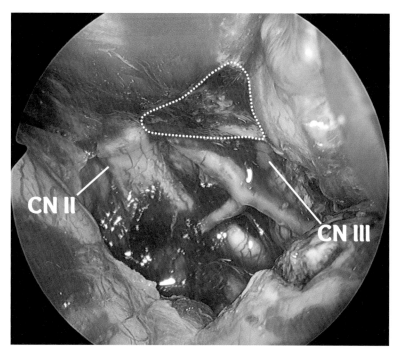

Figure 3-4m. Intradural endoscopic photography taken after tumor removal shows optic nerve (CN II), oculomotor nerve (CN III), and internal carotid artery coursing from the distal dural ring. The dotted area is a dura where the tumor has risen and the anterior clinoid process was. Aided by prior extradural anterior clinoidectomy, the tension which the tumor inflicted on the optic nerve could be relieved before the tumor manipulation.

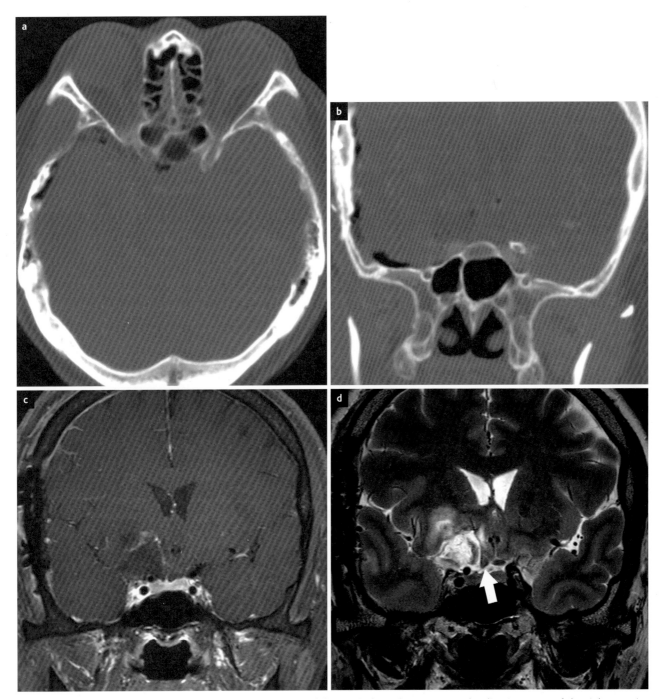

Figure 3-5. (a and b) Post-operative computed tomography with bone windows demonstrates the disappearance of the right anterior clinoid process. (c and d) Post-operative sellar magnetic resonance imaging taken 2 days after surgery shows complete removal of the tumor with relief of adjacent structures. Arrow indicates the right optic nerve, yet is displaced. However, the transactional diameter of the nerve increases as much as that of the contralateral one.

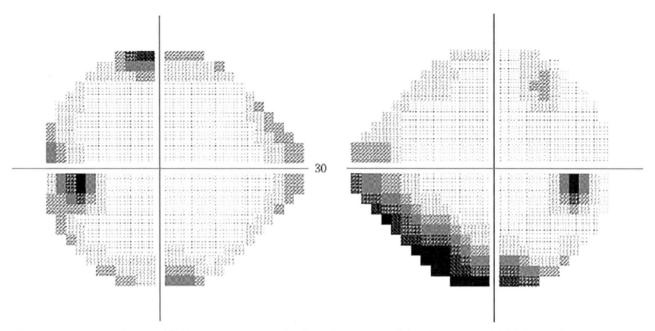

Figure 3-6. Post-operative visual field examination tested 4 days after surgery exhibited an improved field defect of the right eye, of which had had a 360-degree rim-shaped defect.

III. Summary

In the brain, nothing can be more important than the structures of the paraclinoid region. Representatively, the optic nerve and internal carotid artery are the most important structures among them. Besides, encountering those lesions located around the paraclinoid area is also not uncommon to the neurosurgeon. Making more space by moving and visual confirmation before manipulating is essential to preserve those critical structures. intra- or extradurally anterior clinoidectomy has its pros and cons over the opponent's way. Although doing intra- or extradurally would fall according to the characteristics of the lesion, it seems that intradural anterior clinoidectomy is preferred when treating vascular lesions because of necessity in confirming neurovascular structures. In case of the tumor, because making sufficient space to reduce the need for retraction and to achieve early devascularization would be the number one priority, the extradural technique is more likely to be preferred.

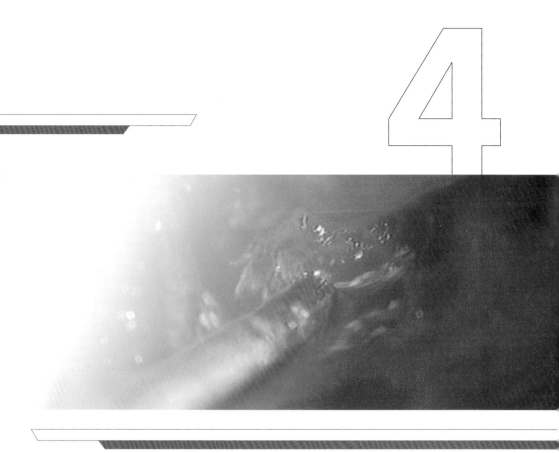

4

CAVERNOUS SINUS APPROACH

Hyuk-Jin Oh M.D., Ph.D., Chang-Ki Hong M.D., Ph.D.
Sung Jin Cho M.D., Ph.D.

I. Introduction

The cavernous sinus is difficult to access surgically due to its complex anatomical structure. Because of the complex structure, damage to blood vessels or nerves occurs, so it is still not an easily accessible structure. The cavernous sinus is a venous structure in the middle cranial fossa that consists of the sella turcica and the dura between the sphenoid bone and the temporal lobe, and where nerves and blood vessels are located. Since Parkinson, the triangular spaces have been widely used as a pathway for surgical approach to the cavernous sinus (**Figure 4-1**).

In this chapter, we demonstrate at the commonly known extradural approach to the cavernous sinus, and the parts mentioned in the anterior clinoidectomy part described first and the anterior petrosal approach described later will be omitted.

1. Preoperative preparation

1) Image studies such as CT and MRI are essential to determine the relationship between the lesion and other cranial structures before surgery. CT helps in the calcification of the lesion and confirmation of the surrounding skull base bony structures. Newly developed proton density MRI images can help distinguish cranial nerves and determine surgical treatment methods.

2) It is necessary to describe the symptoms related to the lesion and understand the condition through cooperation with other departments before and after surgery. Evaluating cranial nerves and blood vessels that pass through or adjacent to the cavernous sinus is essential and can cope with complications or risks that may occur later.

-Extraocular movement (CN II, III, VI) and Visual acuity (CN II).

-Check the cerebral vessel status around tumor through TFCA. The positional relationship between ICA and CS, and the presence or absence of accompanying lesions (cerebral aneurysm, CCF, etc.)

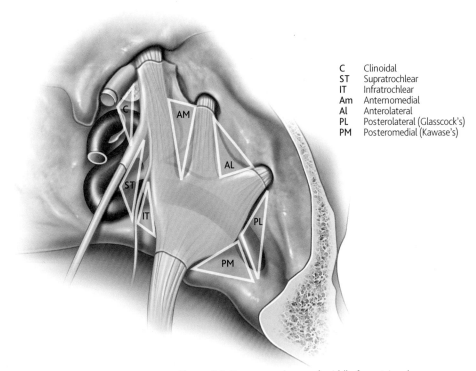

C	Clinoidal
ST	Supratrochlear
IT	Infratrochlear
Am	Anternomedial
Al	Anterolateral
PL	Posterolateral (Glasscock's)
PM	Posteromedial (Kawase's)

Figure 4-1. Cavernous sinus and middle fossa triangles

II. Procedure

1. Anesthesia stage

1) Anesthesia equivalent to general craniotomy is performed, and total intravenous anesthesia is performed in consultation with the anesthesiologist for intraoperative neuromonitoring. SSEP and MEP are monitored for overall monitoring of brain function. Selective neuromonitoring is helped the extraocular muscles to check for damage during surgery.

2) CSF drainage via Lumbar drain may also be performed to prevent intraoperative brain traction injury.

2. Position

The patient position is similar to the pterion approach most familiar to a neurosurgeon. In the supine position, perform neck extension by 10 to 15 degrees and then perform 30 head rotation. Fix the head with a 3-pin head fixator and install neuro-navigation.

3. Skin incision to anterior clinoidectomy

The scalp incision is made within 1cm in front of the tragus from the zygoma position to the midline where the hairline is located. After that, the muscle layer is detached from the bone while preserving the facial nerve using the interfascia approach. Then, an orbitozygomatic approach is performed to perform craniotomy (See Chapter 1). Anterior clinoidectomy was performed for lateral access to the cavernous sinus (See Chapter 3).

4. Extradural stage

After removal of clinoid process, removal of the medial sphenoid wing will help identify the overlying dura. While performing interdural dissection, carefully retract the temporal lobe to expose the foramen rotundum and drilling the upper and lateral surfaces to expose the maxillary nerve (V2) to avoid damage during retraction. The dissection should proceed toward the middle fossa, and the lower part of the temporal bone and the greater wing of the sphenoid bone should be partially removed so that the floor of the middle cranial fossa can be seen directly. Cut the middle meningeal artery from the foramen spinosum and separate the greater and lesser petrosal nerve. Drilling the lateral wall of the foramen ovale to expose the mandibular nerve (V3).

Interdural dissection can be performed to make contact with the outer wall of the cavernous sinus, anteriorly to the petroclinoidal dural fold and posteriorly to the border of the cerebellar tentorium.

Bleeding from the cavernous sinus is venous origin, so hemostasis using Surgicell or flowseal is effective.

Superior approach via Dolenc triangle (Anteromedial triangle)

The dura incision in this approach is made posteriorly after removal of the clinoid process. Although the risk of damaging the cranial nerve passing through the lateral wall is minimal, it is difficult to observe cranial nerves in the lateral wall of the cavernous sinus.

Illustrative case #1

A 74-year-old woman presented with 3rd nerve palsy. MRI demonstrated about 1.7x1.6x1.0cm sized irregular mass with subtle enhancement at left pituitary fossa and lateral side of sella turcica, showing encasement of left ICA and filling left cavernous sinus (**Figure 4-2a**).

She underwent surgery via transsphenoidal approach for pituitary adenoma at another hospital. Tumor removal was planned via Dolenc's triangle.

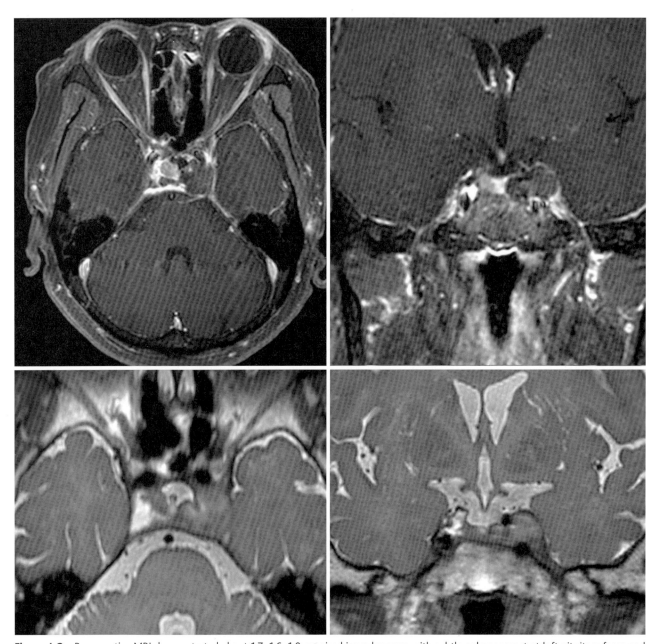

Figure 4-2a. Preoperative MRI demonstrated about 1.7×1.6×1.0 cm sized irregular mass with subtle enhancement at left pituitary fossa and lateral side of sella turcica, showing encasement of left ICA and filling left cavernous sinus. Proton density images are helpful to confirm the relationship between the tumor and surrounding structures in the cavernous sinus.

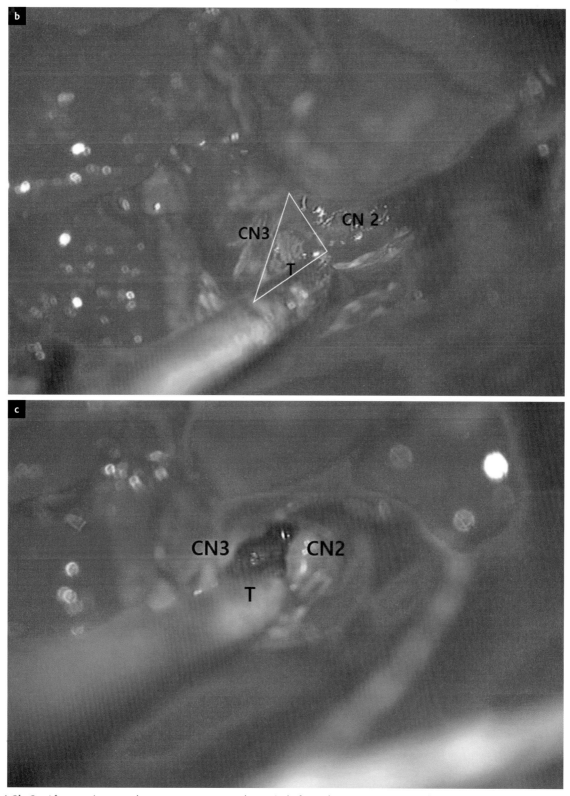

Figure 4-2b, 2c. After craniotomy, the tumor was accessed anteriorly from the cavernous sinus. The tumor was observed in the dolenc triangle.

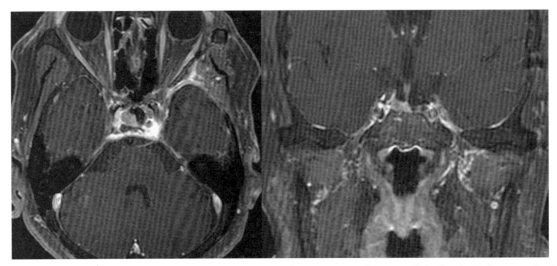

Figure 4-2d. Follow up MRI 1 year after surgery demonstrated complete resection of tumor. Clinically, the 3rd nerve palsy improved gradually after surgery and was fully recovered at 3months.

Lateral approach

Perform interdural dissection to peeled away from V1, V2, and V3. CN3 and CN4 are identified in the anterosuperior lateral wall of the cavernous sinus. The tumor is removed through the infratrochlear triangle (Parkinson's triangle), the anteromedial triangle, and the anterolateral triangle (**Figure 4-3a~f**).

Figure 4-3a~f.

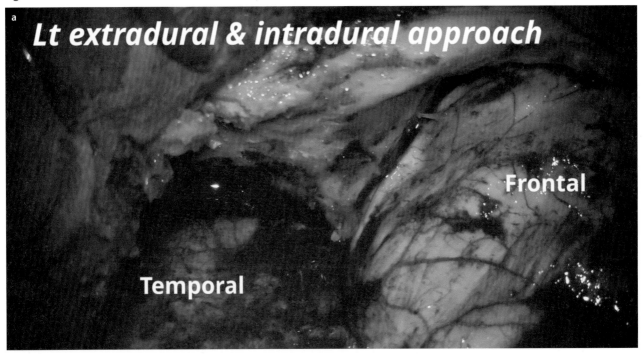

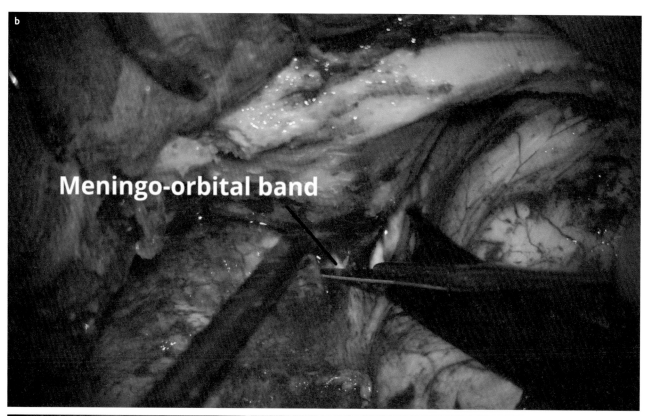

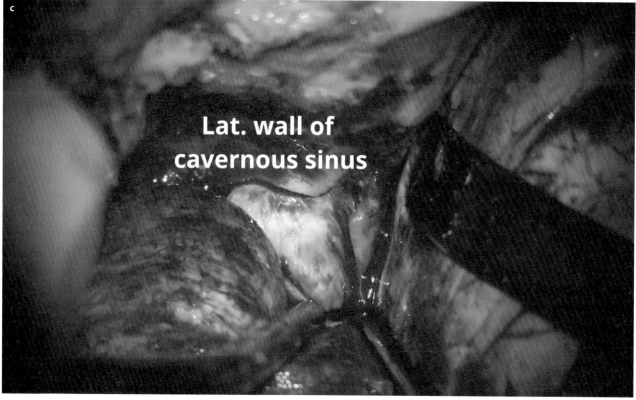

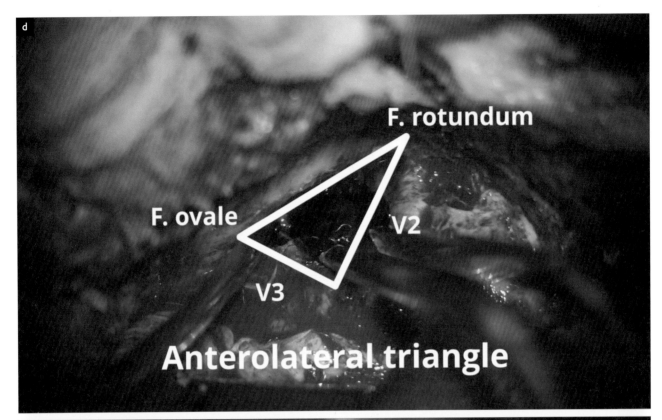

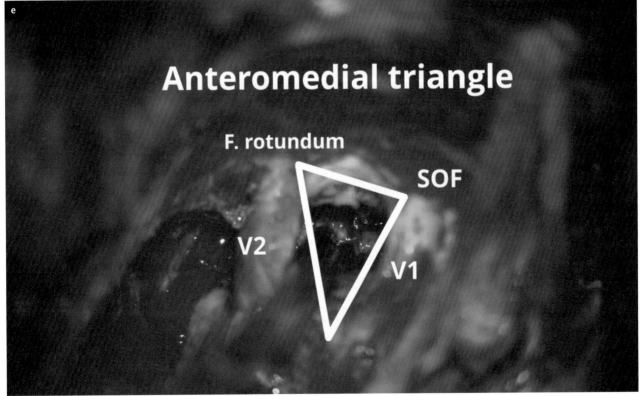

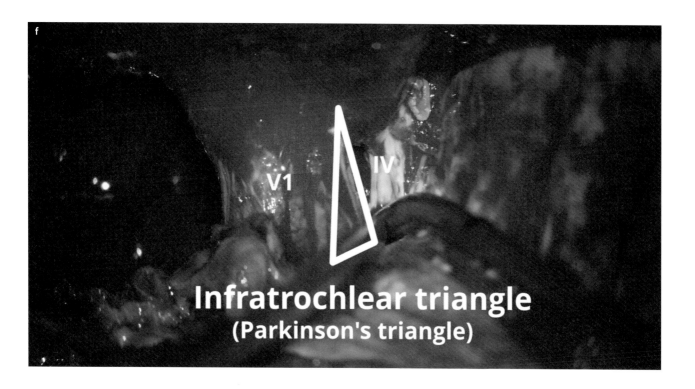

Illustrative case #2

A 29-year-old woman presented with right facial pain. MRI demonstrated 2.4×1.7×1.8 cm sized round well marginated enhancing lesion in right cavernous sinus (Figure 4-4a).

Tumor removal was planned via cavernous sinus approach.

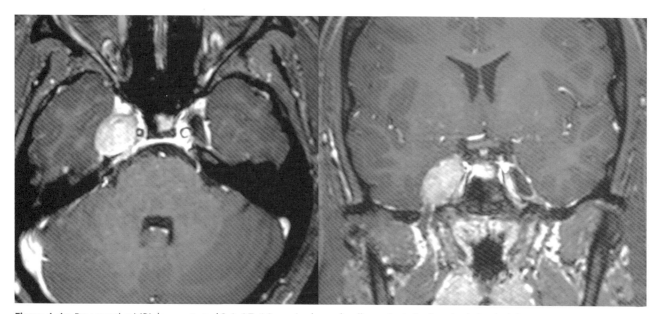

Figure 4-4a. Preoperative MRI demonstrated 2.4×1.7×1.8 cm sized round well marginated enhancing lesion in right cavernous sinus. The tumor showed prominent enhancement in the T1 contrast enhancement image, which was confined to the middle fossa.

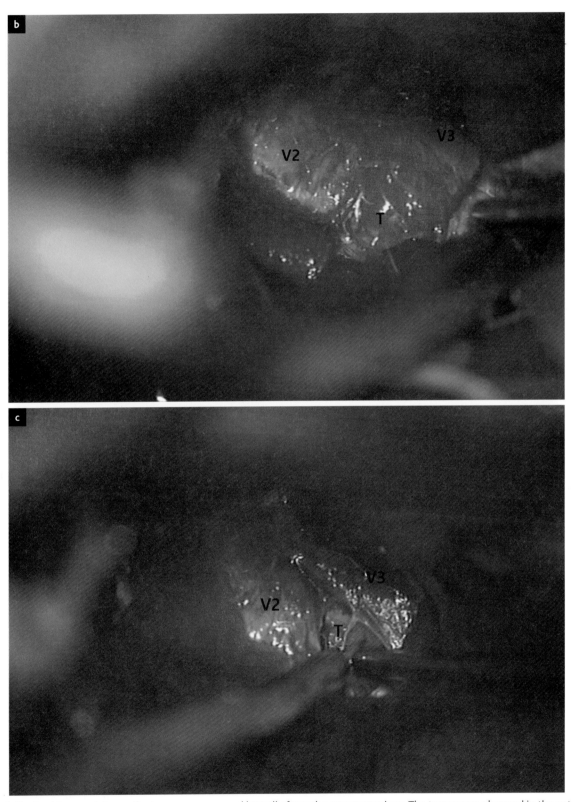

Figure 4-4b, 4c. After craniotomy, the tumor was accessed laterally from the cavernous sinus. The tumor was observed in the anterolateral triangle.

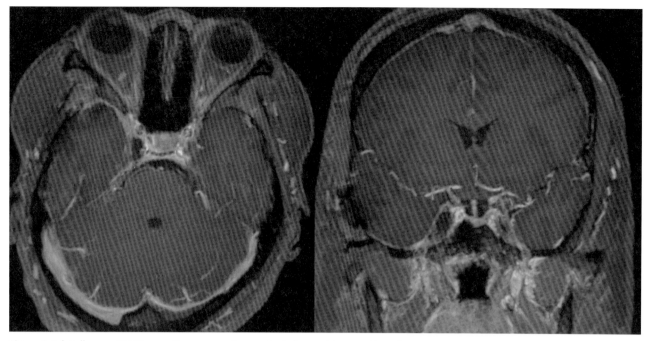

Figure 4-4d. Follow up MRI 1 year after surgery demonstrated complete resection of tumor.

III. Tip & Summary

1. In order to access the cavernous sinus, orbitozygomatic craniotomy can be added depending on the position to be accessed after the frontemporal craniotomy.

2. One of the most important techniques in the extradural approach is to find the dissecting plane between the dura mater of the temporal lobe and the lateral wall of CS. It may be easier to dissect using a blunt dissector than using a sharp microsurgical instrument.

3. If bleeding occurs during dissection of the cavernous sinus and then hemostasis using bipolar, damage to the cranial nerve occurs. Effective hemostatic can be achieved by applying surgicell or flowseal and waiting.

4. If the space from which the tumor is removed after surgery is large, CSF leakage may occur, so a fat graft should be considered.

5. The dura mater should be sutured as much as possible, and tachocomb or artificial dura substitute material should not be trusted too much.

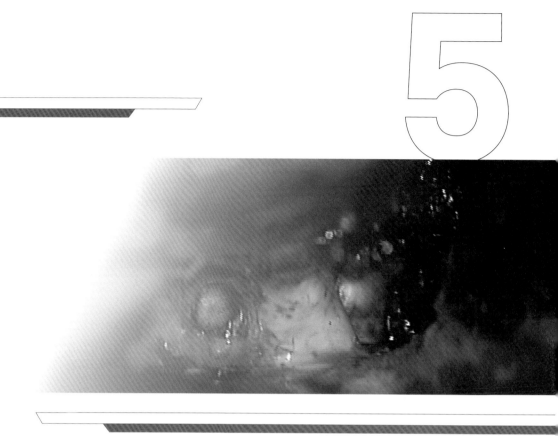

ANTERIOR PETROSAL APPROACH

Chang-Ki Hong M.D., Ph.D.

I. Introduction

The anterior petrosal approach is used for the radical resection of small and medium-size tumors originating above the internal auditory canal. The approach allows to resect the dura covering the anterior petrous bone as well as the adjacent tentorium and gives us access to tumor coursing into Meckel's cave. Surgical access to the anterior of brainstem represents a formidable neurosurgical challenge because of the region's anatomic complexity, depth, and concentration of critical neurovascular structures.

The goal of the anterior petrosal approach is to expose the anterior and anterolateral aspects of the up-per third of the brainstem. The main advantage of the anterior petrosal approach is the direct access allowed to tumors attached to the clivus through a corridor created on the petrous apex.

II. Patient positioning and skin incision

Before positioning the patient, we place a lumbar drain. Cerebrospinal fluid (CSF) drainage through the lumbar drain is imperative in avoiding temporal lobe injury during the lobe's extradural retraction. Often 40 to 60 cc of CSF is drained gradually until the lobe

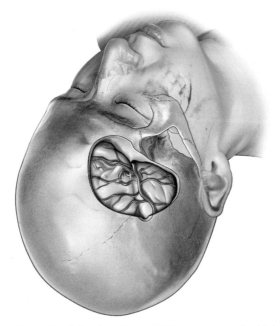

Figure 5-1. Patient's head position with the zygoma as the highest point on the operative field. The vertex of the patient's head is tilted slightly toward the floor. This maneuver maximizes the effect of gravity retraction on the temporal lobe. Curvilinear scalp incision. It starts immediately posterior to the ear and finally descends to the level of the zygomatic arch, about 1 to 2 centimeters in front of the tragus. The curvilinear incision mobilizes the muscle effectively away from the operative working zone.

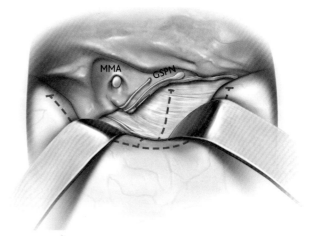

Figure 5-2. The dura over the floor of the anterior aspect of the middle fossa is now generously elevated. The middle meningeal artery (red arrow), entering through the foramen spinosum, is identified along the anterior aspect of the bone exposure. The artery must be coagulated on its dural side and transected. Next, I pack the foramen with bone wax and oxidized cellulose. Stripping of the dura anteriorly must stop at this point to avoid direct injury to the greater (GSPN)(yellow arrow) and lesser superficial petrosal nerves (LSPN), leading potentially to dry eyes. Inadvertent traction on the GSPN will also place the facial nerve at risk. The surgeon can minimize the risk of this type of injury by lifting the dura in a posterior-to-anterior direction.

is completely mobilized for adequate exposure of the middle fossa floor. Abdominal preparation is also important procedure for harvesting fat grafts used for dural closure.

The patient is positioned supine on the operating table. A shoulder roll is placed under the patient's contralateral shoulder and the head rotated until the sagittal suture is parallel to or minimally angled from the floor. If the patient has a supple neck, he or she can tolerate up from 60 to 80 degrees of rotation to ensure sphenoid ridge parallel to the floor.

A myofascial cuff may be left on the bone to facilitate closure. For the horseshoe incision, the flap is reflected inferiorly with fishhooks; enough muscle dissection should be completed until the posterior root of the zygomatic arch is clearly visible. The operator must take care not to dissect so low as to violate the mandibular joint or external auditory canal.

After the craniotomy flap is elevated, the remaining base of the temporal squama is reduced flush with the floor of the middle fossa. This goal can be accomplished using rongeurs or a drill with a side-cutting burr. Air cells are often exposed at this step of the operation and must be thoroughly obliterated with bone wax to prevent creation of a CSF fistula. The superior edge of the zygomatic arch may also be drilled to provide an unobstructed view of the floor of the middle fossa, but this is rarely necessary.

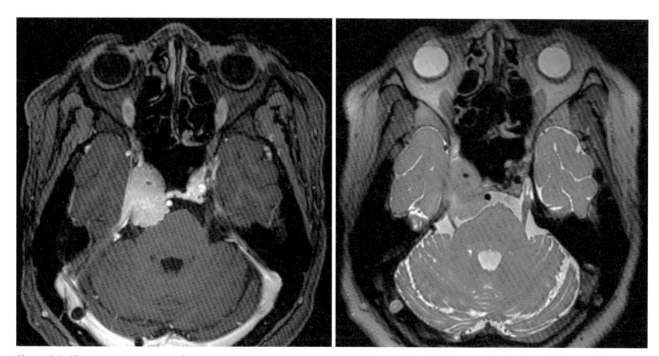

Figure 5-3. The patient is 65-year-old woman who presented with trigeminal neuralgia. MRI shows petroclival meningioma with cavernous sinus invasion. Trigeminal nerve is displaced laterally.

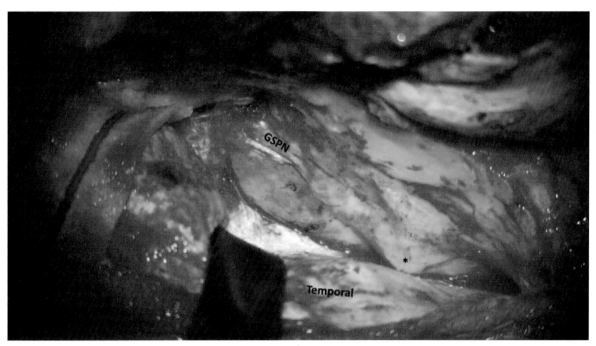

Figure 5-4. Exposure of Kawase's triangle. With the dura completely elevated to the level of the petrous ridge, the landmarks of Kawase's quadrilateral are clearly visible: laterally, the GSPN posteriorly, the arcuate eminence; anteriorly, the posterior edge of the V3; and medially, the petrous ridge.

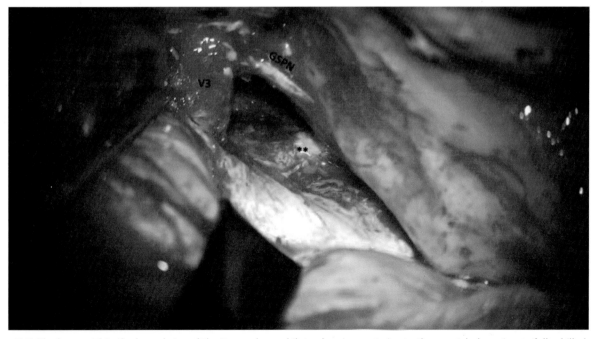

Figure 5-5. The bone within the boundaries of the Kawase's quadrilateral region, anterior to the meatal plane, is carefully drilled using a rough diamond burr along with abundant irrigation to prevent thermal damage to the underlying structures such as internal auditory canal(**). The basic technique is to core out the central portion of the bony apex and later, using curettes, remove the thin shell of bone from the dura. All of the bone between the V3 anteriorly, the ICA and the cochlea laterally, and the superior semicircular canal and the IAC posteriorly is drilled away until the dura of the posterior fossa is reached, thereby completing the anterior transpetrosal osteotomy.

III. Intradural procedure

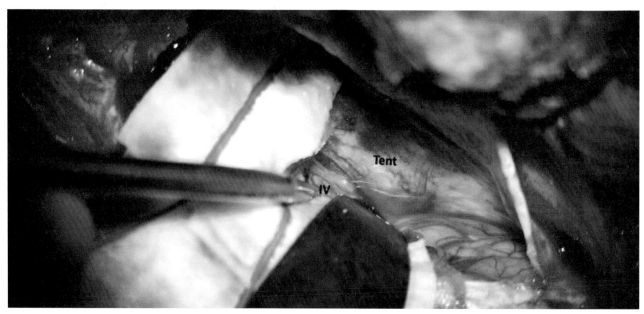

Figure 5-6. The dural opening is planned as a T-shaped incision. The first incision is made along the basal temporal dura parallel to the inferior edge of the craniotomy. The second cut is perpendicular to the first, crossing the superior petrosal sinus into the posterior fossa dura. The superior petrosal sinus is then ligated using a Dural clip and the dural incisions connected. The posterior limb of the incision must be carefully completed to ensure that the trochlear nerve and vein of Labbé are not injured. The tentorium is then transected posteriorly to the point where cranial nerve V enters the dura. The operator should also be especially careful during these dural incisions to protect the trochlear and trigeminal nerve-it can easily be inadvertently transected due to its displacement by the true petroclival meningioma as it enters the Meckel cave at the porus trigeminus.
IV; trochlear nerve, Tent; tentorium.

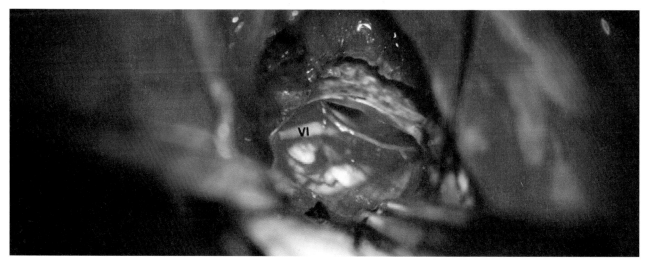

Figure 5-7. Right sided anterior petrosectomy: intradural exposure and operative field. The end result of the procedure is a generous anterolateral view of the structures of the posterior fossa through a middle fossa corridor. A Petroclival meningioma can be readily resected through this corridor. Cranial V is the center of the operative corridor in this approach and can be easily injured during dural opening because trigeminal nerve is displaced laterally by the tumor.

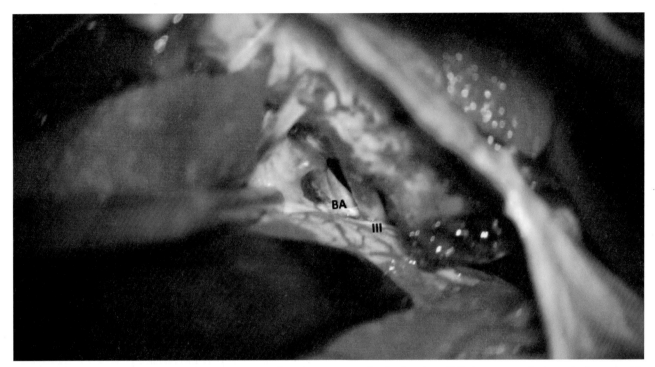

Figure 5-8. anterior-superior view. Oculomotor nerve and Basilar artery can be displaced medially large petroclival meningioma. In this case, the oculomotor nerve is not affected. But tumor is invaded into oculomotor triangle.

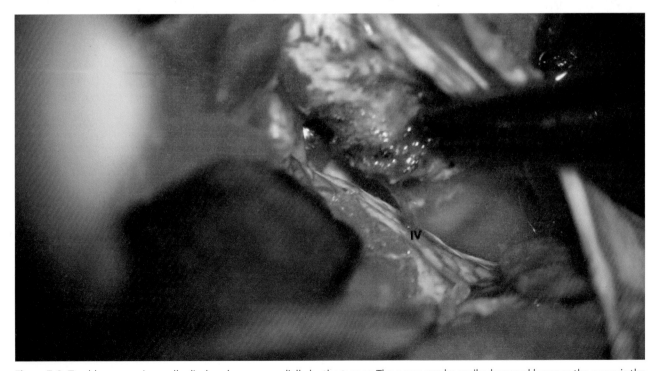

Figure 5-9. Trochlear nerve is usually displaced supero-medially by the tumor. The nerve can be easily damaged because the nerve is the thinnest and longest. Furthermore the nerve is adhered to the tumor and it is hard to find the trochlear nerve.

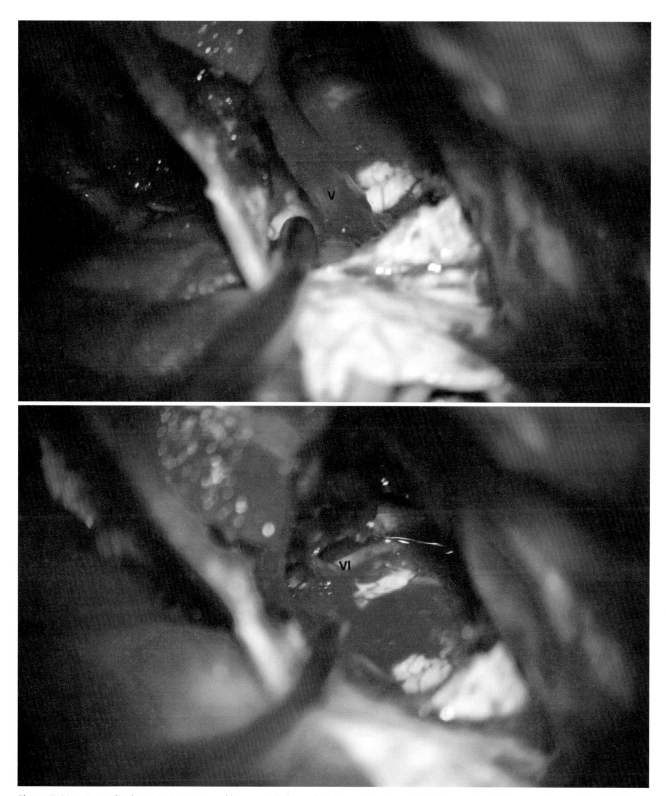

Figure 5-10. A Petroclival meningioma is readily resected through this corridor. Cranial V is the center of the operative corridor in this approach.

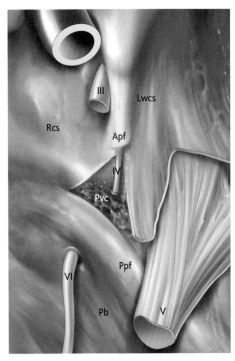

Figure 5-11. Visualization of the abducens nerve (VI) after removing the tumor. The nerve arises from the ponto-medullary junction from a single trunk or two distinct trunks. The nerve leaves the posterior fossa by piercing the meningeal dura over the clivus approximately 1 cm below and medial to the trigeminal root. The relationships between Dorello's canal and inferior petrosal sinus are very closed. For the first few millimeters of its intradural course, this nerve is sheathed by the arachnoid and bathed in CSF. It can be deduced that the petroclival portion of the abducens nerve does not belong to the extradural space. This is an important observation because, at the level of the petrous apex, it twists round horizontally under the Gruber's ligament to pass over the dorsal and lateral surface of the internal carotid artery as it enters the posterior cavernous sinus. The basilar artery is exposed over a little more than one centimeter as well as the AICA from its origin as far as the ventral part of its loop.

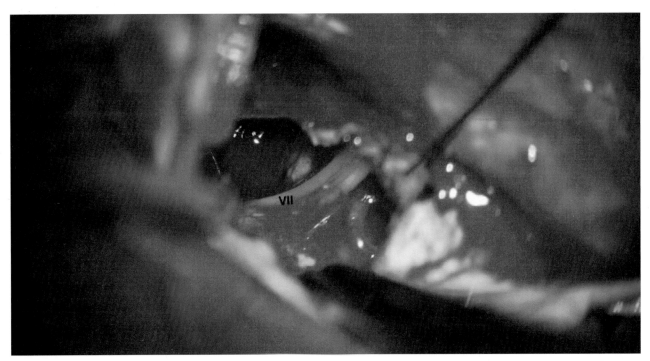

Figure 5-12. VII seven-eight complex; It runs in an almost frontal plane as it crosses the cistern of the pontocerebellar angle (cerebellopontine cistern). In our case, the AICA crosses the nervous bundle by its dorsal face, the loop being fixed by the dura mater above the porus. This neurovascular structure transversally crosses the cerebellopontine angle and is protected by the arachnoid sheath of its individual cistern. Even though it is outside the petroclival region, it is exposed in the surgical field laid open by a number of common approaches to the PCR. Tumors originating from the PCR usually push the cerebellopontine cistern and its contents backwards.

IV. Closure

If petrosal air cells have been opened, they should be covered with two or three layers of fibrin sealant patches. Primary dural closure is obviously impossible in this area and alternative methods are needed. Collagen based dural graft is used to cover the dural defect. The surgical cavity can be filled with abdominal fat. The fat is also one of the excellent barriers against CSF leakage. Strips of adipose tissue are placed across the dural opening to seal the dural defect. Bone flap is replaced and secured using miniplates, and the rest of closure is conducted in the standard fashion. If postoperative rhinorrhea or wound CSF collection is encountered, a lumbar drain is continued for 3-4 days.

REFERENCES

1. Cho CW, Al-Mefty O. Combined petrosal approach to petroclival meningiomas. Neurosurgery 2002;51(3):708-18.

2. Day JD, Fukushima T, Giannotta SL. Microanatomical study of the extradural middle fossa approach to the petroclival and posterior cavernous sinus region: description of the rhomboid construct. Neurosurgery 1994;34(6):1009-16.

3. de Oliveira E, Rhoton AL Jr, Peace D. Microsurgical anatomy of the region of the foramen magnum. Surg Neurol 1985;24(3):293-352.

4. Destrieux C, Velut S, Kakou MK, Lefrancq T, Arbeille B, Santini JJ. A new concept in Dorello's canal microanatomy: the petroclival venous confluence. J Neurosurg 1997;87(1):67-72.

5. Dolenc VV, Skrap M, Sustersic J, Skrbec M, Morina A. A transcavernous-transsellar approach to the basilar tip aneurysms. Br J Neurosurg 1987;1(2):251-9.

6. Fournier HD, Mercier P, Menei P, Alhayek G, Guy G. Transpetrosal approaches to the clivus. Surgical anatomy, pretentions and limit. Neurochirurgie 1995;41(1):6-28.

7. Fournier HD, Mercier P. A limited anterior petrosectomy with preoperative embolisation of the inferior petrosal sinus for ventral brainstem tumor removal. Surg Neurol 2000;54:10-8.

8. Fukushima T, Day JD, Hirahara K. Extradural total petrous apex resection with trigeminal translocation for improved exposure of the posterior cavernous sinus and petroclival region. Skull Base Surg 1996;6(2):95-103.

9. Hakuba A, Nishimura S, Inoue Y. Transpetrosal-transtentorial approach and its application in the therapy of retrochiasmatic craniopharyngiomas. Surg Neurol 1985;24(4):405-15.

10. House WF, Hitselberger WE, Horn KL. The middle fossa transpetrous approach to the anterior-superior cerebellopontine angle. Am J Otol 1986;7(1):1-4.

11. Kawase T, Shiobara R, Toya S. Anterior transpetrosal transtentorial approach for sphenopetroclival meningiomas: surgical method and results in 10 patients. Neurosurgery 1991;28:869-76.

12. Kawase T, Toya S, Shiobara R, Mine T. Transpetrosal approach for aneurysms of the lower basilar artery. J Neurosurg 1985;63(6):857-61.

13. Matsushima T, Rhoton AL Jr, de Oliveira E, Peace D. Microsurgical anatomy of the veins of the posterior fossa. J Neurosurg 1983;59(1):63-105.

14. Mickey B, Close L, Schaefer S, Samson D. A combined frontotemporal and lateral infratemporal fossa approach to the skull base. J Neurosurg 1988;68(5):678-83.

15. Ozveren MF, Uchida K, Aiso S, Kawase T. Meningovenous structures of the petroclival region: clinical importance for surgery and intravascular surgery. Neurosurgery 2002;50(4):829-36.

16. Rhoton AL Jr. Microsurgery of the internal acoustic meatus. Surg Neurol 1974;2(5):311-8.

17. Rhoton AL, Hardy DG, Chambers SM. Microsurgical anatomy and dissections of the sphenoid bone, cavernous sinus and sellar region. Surg Neurol 1979;12(1):63-104.

18. Sekhar LN, Janecka IP, Jones NF. Subtemporal-infratemporal and basal subfrontal approach to extensive cranial base tumors. Acta Neurochir (Wien) 1988;92:83-92.

19. Sekhar LN, Schramm VL Jr, Jones NF. Subtemporal preauricular infratemporal fossa approach to large lateral and posterior cranial base neoplasms. J Neurosurg 1987;67:488-99.

20. Sen CN, Sekhar LN. The subtemporal and preauricular infratemporal approach to intradural structures ventral to the brain stem. J Neurosurg 1990;73(3):345-54.

21. Sen C, Chen CS, Post KD. Microsurgical anatomy of the skull base and approaches to the cavernous sinus. New York: Thieme;1997.p.42

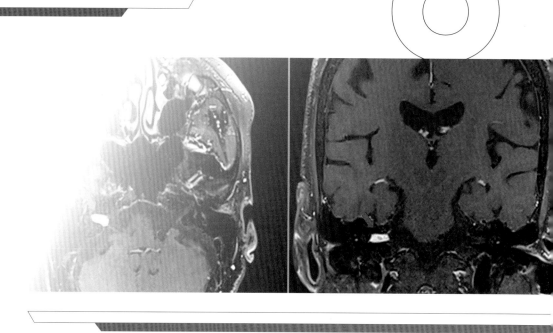

6

MIDDLE CRANIAL FOSSA APPROACH TO INTERNAL AUDITORY CANAL

Sung-Il Nam M.D., Ph.D.

I. Introduction

The middle cranial fossa approach was first introduced in 1892, but was not used for a while due to the limited knowledge and clinical risk of the time. This middle fossa approach was used in earnest since the introduction of the operating microscope by the W. F. House in the 1960s. In the past, the purpose of surgery of acoustic tumor was to remove the tumor and preserve life. However, due to the early detection of tumors due to the recent development of gadolinium-enhanced magnetic resonance imaging (MRI), the preservation of hearing as well as the function of the facial nerve has come to be considered important.

1. Advantages

1) It shows the highest hearing preservation rate compared to other approaches.
2) The frequency of headaches after surgery is low.
3) It provides complete exposure of the contents of the internal auditory canal, allowing removal of laterally placed tumors.

2. Disadvantages

1) It is difficult to apply to large tumors
2) It is technically difficult due to lack of strong landmarks and limited exposure.

3. Indications

1) Intracanalicular tumor with a cerebellopontine angle extension of less than 5mm and serviceable hearing (speech reception threshold>50dB, speech discrimination score>70%, these indications should be individualized according to the patient's needs)
2) Facial schwannoma of the internal auditory canal and the geniculate ganglion
3) Facial nerve decompression in Bell's palsy or Ramsay Hunt syndrome

4. Contraindications

1) Older than 65years
2) Inflammation of the temporal bone, such as chronic otitis media

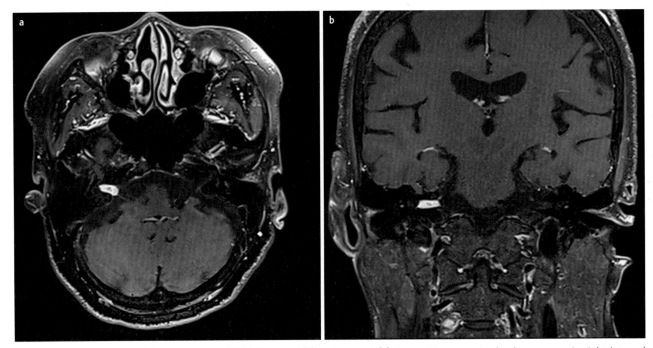

Figure 6-1. T1 weighted gadolinium-enhanced MRI. The axial (a) and coronal (b) shows 11×4 mm sized enhance mass in right internal auditory canal.

5. Preoperative considerations

1) Audiometric testing within a few days of surgery
2) Magnetic resonance imaging and CT scan of the temporal bone
3) Preoperative VNG (videonystagmography) may predict tumor origin and hearing preservation. Caloric test, VEMP test and video head impulse test needed.
4) Measurement of serum electrolytes, blood urea nitrogen, creatine, complete blood count, prothrombin time and partial thromboplastin time
5) Chest X-ray and EKG if indicated
6) Informed consent detailing possible complications, including hearing loss, facial paralysis, dizziness, intracranial hematoma, infection, meningitis, aphasia, stroke and death

II. Case

A 58-year-old male patient presented with dizziness, gradual right hearing loss, and tinnitus for 2 months. In the video head impulse test (vHIT), overt and covert saccades appeared in right side, and vHIT gain decreased in right side (**Figure 6-2b**). The caloric tes showed 50.6% canal paresis in right ear (**Figure 6-2c**). Pure tone audiometry revealed mild sensorineural hearing loss on the right (**Figure 6-2a**). An MRI scan shows 11 × 4 mm sized enhanced mass in right internal auditory canal (**Figure 6-1**). The tumor was removed via the middle cranial fossa approach.

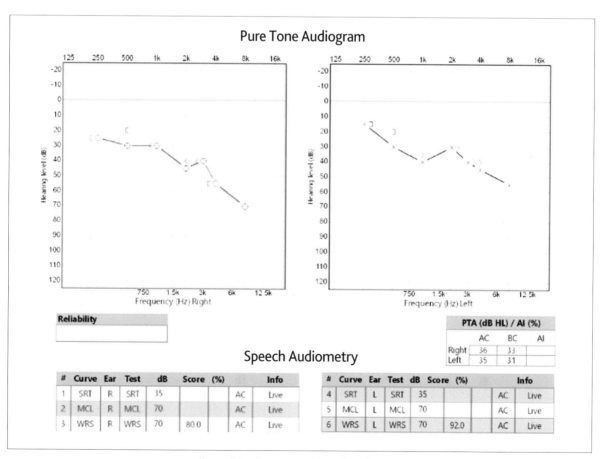

Figure 6-2a. Puretone and speech audiometry.

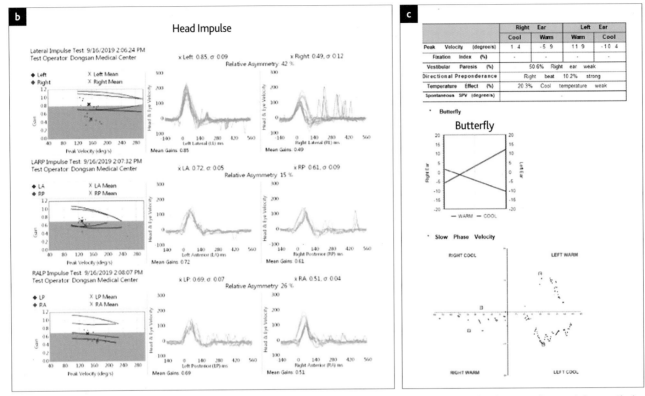

Figure 6-2b,c. video head impulse test (b) and caloric test (c) shows decreased right side vestibular function due to right vestibular schwannoma.

III. Procedure

1. Skin incision is commonly used in two methods :
1) 'ㄷ'-shaped incision method. Make a 6 × 8 cm skin incision in a 'ㄷ'-shape with a base from the upper part of the auricle to the rear (**Figure 6-3a**). Ligation of the superficial temporal artery can be avoided.
2) 'S'-shaped incision method. Incision starts in the zygomatic root, pretragal area and extends to 7 to 8 cm superiorly. In a gently anterior curving fashion (**Figure 6-3b**)
2. The flap of skin and subcutaneous tissue is elevated, then temporalis fascia and muscle are divided using monopolar diathermy. It is useful to harvest the temporal fascia.
3. A quadrangular 4×5 cm craniotomy is performed (**Figure 6-4**). The craniotomy located approximately two thirds anterior and one third posterior to the external auditory canal. The craniotomy begins with a burr hole and then using cutting and diamond burrs. The lower edge of the craniotomy should be at the level of the base of the zygoma, so that it is approximately at the level of the floor of the middle cranial fossa.
4. The craniotomy flap is carefully dissected from the underlying dura using a dissector to avoid tearing the dura The flap is removed and placed in wet gauze.
5. Elevation of the dura from the superior surface of temporal bone is performed under a surgical microscope. Because it is the most delicate step during the operation. Dural elevation should be carried from posterior to anterior. When the dura is elevated anteriorly, the greater superficial petrosal nerve (GSPN) is encountered. In approximately 10~15% of cases, the geniculate ganglion (GG) is dehiscent.

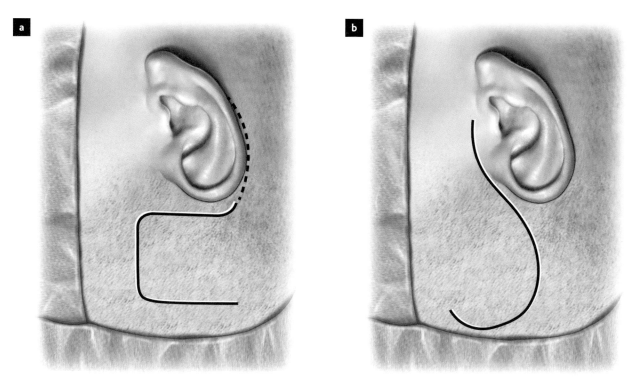

Figure 6-3. The skin incision is made as shown. ' ⊏ '-shaped incision method (a), 'S'-shaped incision method (b)

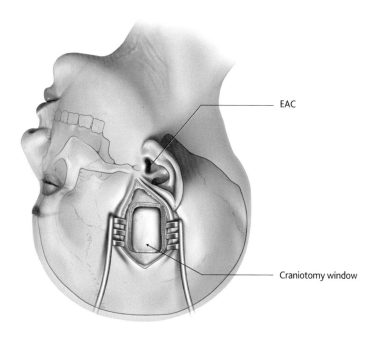

EAC

Craniotomy window

Figure 6-4. The craniotomy is performed in the squamous portion using a drill.

63

The GSPN is located on the medial side of the middle meningeal artery and passes parallel to the apex of the petrous.

6. The initial landmark is the middle meningeal artery, which marks the anterior extent of the dissection. Frequently venous bleeding is encountered from this area, and it can be controlled with bipolar coagulation, Surgicel, gelfoam and thrombin (**Figure 6-5**). Also, the arcuate eminence and greater superficial petrosal nerve (GSPN) are identified.

7. When the dura has been elevated, the retractor is applied (**Figure 6-6**).

8. Four different methods can be used to identify the internal auditory canal.

1) The House method (**Figure 6-7a**). The internal auditory canal is found in the fundus area. Since the ampulla of the superior semicircular canal and the basal turn of the cochlea are very close to this area, it is necessary to pay close attention not to damage these structures and the labyrinth segment of the

facial nerve during the drilling process.

2) Fisch method (**Figure 6-7b**). Using the largest diamond burr, drill the back and top of the arcuate eminence to find the superior semicircular canal first. Once the blue line is identified, the internal auditory is found at an angle of 60 degrees anteriorly.

3) Garcia Ibanez method (**Figure 6-7c**). After finding the GSPN and the superior semicircular canal, the internal auditory canal corresponds approximately to the line bisecting the angle made by the arcuate eminence and GSPN. Drilling is started medially at the level of the porus of internal auditory canal.

4) Method using ossicles (**Figure 6-7d**). This is a method of estimating the vertical crest of the IAC after finding the ossicles by exposing the tegmen of the middle ear cavity.

Once the IAC identified, three quarters of the canal circumference (270°) is skeletonized, leaving a only thin shell of bone.

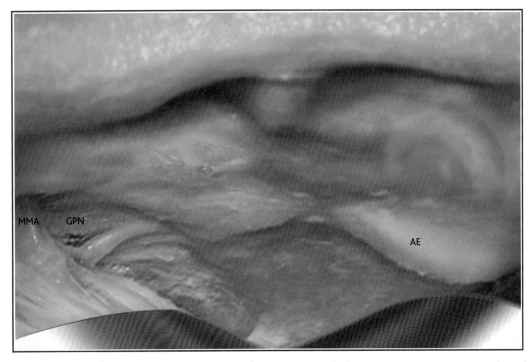

Figure 6-5. The Following landmarks should be identified: the arcuate eminence (AE), the middle meningeal artery (MMA), the greater superficial petrosal nerve (GPN).

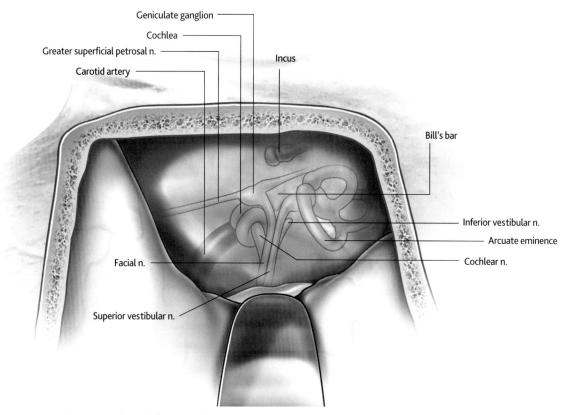

Figure 6-6. The middle cranial fossa retractor has been applied to the elevated dura.

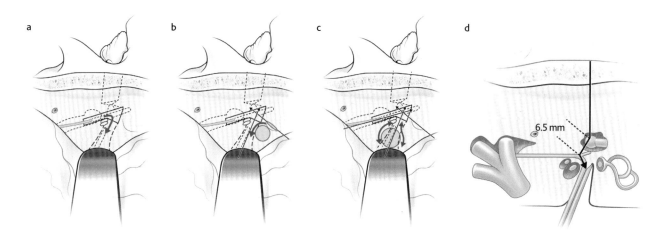

Figure 6-7. Four different methods can be used to identify the internal auditory canal.

9. Drilling is continued laterally to expose the entire length of IAC. To avoid injury to IAC, the drill should be moved parallel to the IAC (**Figure 6-8**).

10. After the IAC is identified, the posterior fossa dura can be opened with Beaver knife to release the cerebrospinal fluid. After opening the mater of the IAC

and identify the Bill's bar, check the facial nerve and the superior vestibular nerve (**Figure 6-9**).

11. Seperation of the tumor is initially performed at the Bill's bar, but all dissections proceed from medial to lateral along the facial nerve. The arachnoid is divided, and the margin of the facial nerve is identi-

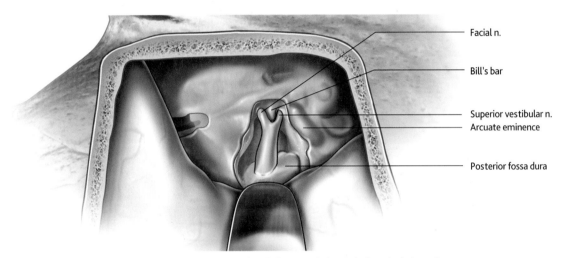

Facial n.

Bill's bar

Superior vestibular n.
Arcuate eminence

Posterior fossa dura

Figure 6-8. The internal auditory canal is skeletonized through the whole length.

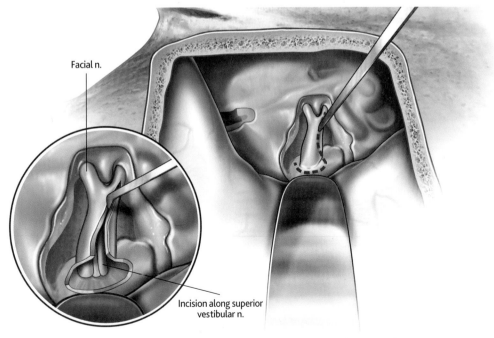

Facial n.

Incision along superior vestibular n.

Figure 6-9. Dura of the internal auditory canal is opened.

fied. The facial-vestibular connection is sharply cut. Tumor removal is performed from a medial to lateral direction to avoid injury of the cochlear nerve and blood supply (**Figure 6-10**). The outermost part of the anterior inferior cerebellar artery can be located anywhere in the cerebellopontine angle or at the base of the IAC, it should be carefully identified

and separated from the tumor.

12. After removal of the tumor, the surgical field is thoroughly cleaned, and abdominal fat is used to fill the defect in the IAC. The incision site is closed. A mastoid compressive dressing is maintained for 2 days postoperatively (**Figure 6-11**).

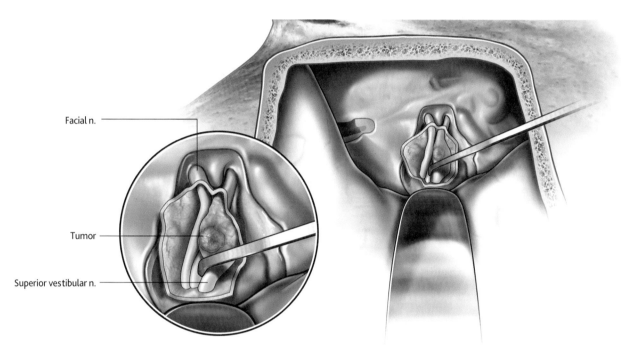

Facial n.

Tumor

Superior vestibular n.

Figure 6-10. An intracanalicular tumor is seperated from the facial and cochlear nerves.

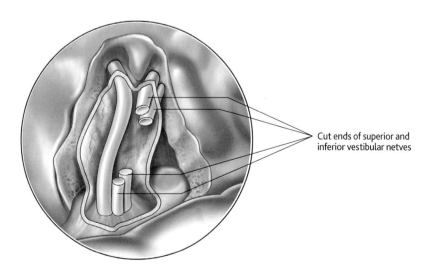

Cut ends of superior and inferior vestibular netves

Figure 6-11. Cut ends of superior and inferior vestibular nerves are shown after removal of the tumor.

67

IV. Tip and Summary

1. The middle cranial fossa approach allows hearing preservation as well as complete exposure of the entire length of the internal auditory canal, and provides excellent access of the removal of intra-canalicular tumors.

2. The craniotomy should be performed at the level of the root of the zygoma. This will improve the surgical field and reduce the temporal lobe retraction.

3. The IAC is located approximately on the same axis as the external auditory canal; this relationship is useful in orienting the surgical field.

4. Identifying the IAC is the most important and difficult process, so should be familiar with all the different methods to find the IAC and be able to operate according to the situation.

5. In order to minimize the injury to the facial nerve, the facial nerve should be separated from the facial nerve, rather than from the tumor

6. The IAC dura is opened posteriorly in order to avoid injuring the facial nerve.

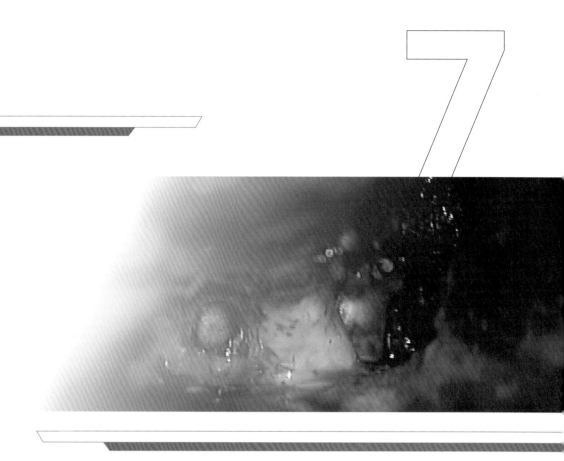

7

TRANSLABYRINTHINE APPROACH

Beom Cho Jun M.D., Ph.D., Ki-Hong Chang M.D., Ph.D.

I. Introduction

The approach to the internal auditory canal (IAC) through the lateral temporal bone is obscured by labyrinths. The removal of labyrinth to expose the neural compartment in the IAC is the main concept of this procedure.

Translabyrinthine approach shows a wide field of surgical view of temporal bone, therefore most of the critical structures of temporal bone could be identified and managed.

In particular, the facial nerve pathway could be identified from the segments of IAC to the fallopian canal of the mastoid with this approach. Therefore, it is also used as a technique for exploring the facial nerve in case of traumatic facial nerve paralysis or facial nerve schwannoma.

Generally, this approach is applied for the removal of tumors in patients with non-serviceable hearing due to growing vestibular schwannoma involving the IAC.

It could also be used for other tumors in the cerebellopontine angle (CPA). These include meningiomas, epidermoids, glomus tumors, and choroid plexus papillomas.

- Pre-operative preparation or check points

1. imaging study

2. Functional study of hearing and balance

Consensus of non-serviceable hearing

Some centers adhere to a 50-50 rule in which the hearing is serviceable if the pure tone average is 50 dB or less, and the speech discrimination score is 50% to 100%. Other centers use the 30-70 rule in which hearing is serviceable if the pure tone average is 30 dB or less and the speech discrimination score is 70% to 100%.

II. Procedure

1. General anesthesia and preparation

After satisfactory anesthesia is induced, the patient receives an oro-gastric tube, a foley catheter, recording needle electrodes into the facial musculature with supine position. Turning the patient head to the opposite site, The operative sites at the ear, scalp, and neck, as well as the fat harvest site in the left, lower quadrant, are then outlined with adhesive drapes.

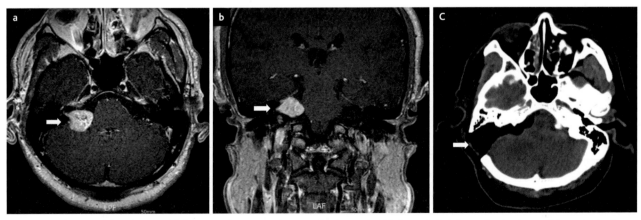

Figure 7-1. The axial (a) and coronal (b) image of preoperative T1 Gd enhanced MRI shows 2.0×1.8 cm sized enhanced mass in the internal auditory canal and cerebellopontine angle. The postoperative brain CT (c) shows bony defect and fat infiltration after right translabyrinthine approach.

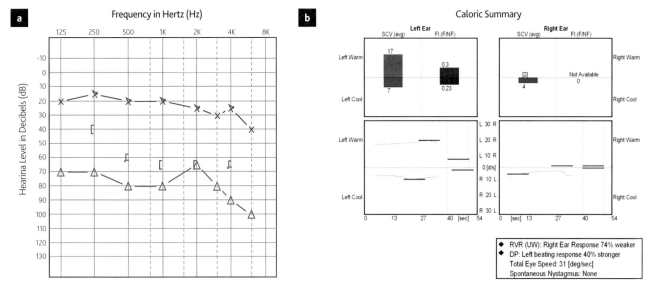

Figure 7-2. Pure tone audiometry (a) and caloric test (b) shows decreased hearing and vestibular function due to compression of vestibular schwannoma.

2. Skin incision and complete mastoidectomy with mastoid facial nerve identify

A retro-auricular incision is performed 4 cm posteriorly from the auricular sulcus. Complete mastoidectomy should be performed to fully expose the internal auditory canal, including the tumor. During mastoidectomy, the mastoid segments of the facial nerve are identified and preserved (**Figure 7-3**).

3. Thinning of Sigmoid Sinus

Bone is removed from the middle and presigmoid posterior fossa dura. It helps sigmoid sinus be more exposed in the operation fields. The sigmoid sinus is then decompressed with a bony island of bone (the Bill bar) to protect it as drilling proceeds medially. This procedure secures a sufficient space of sinodural angle, posterior fossa dura and jugular bulb. This enables them to supply the room to drill for the Contour of IAC (**Figure 7-3**).

4. Identify Semicircular canal and Endolymphatic sac

Complete removal of the air cells in the mastoid cavity reveals the contour of the labyrinth. The lateral semicircular canal (SCC) is located at the bottom of the mastoid antrum. The endolymphatic sac is located 60 degrees inside the point, where the Donaldson line meets the sigmoid sinus (**Figure 7-3**). The endolymphatic duct from the sac runs inside the SCC and connects with the vestibule.

5. Labyrinthectomy

The ampulla of superior SCC is preserved during labyrinthectomy because the ampulla branch of the superior vestibular nerve becomes the landmark for the finding of IAC. Labyrinthectomy proceeds in the order of lateral SCC, posterior SCC, and superior SCC. In particular, the subarcuate artery runs in the center of the concentric circles of the superior SCC (**Figure 7-4**).

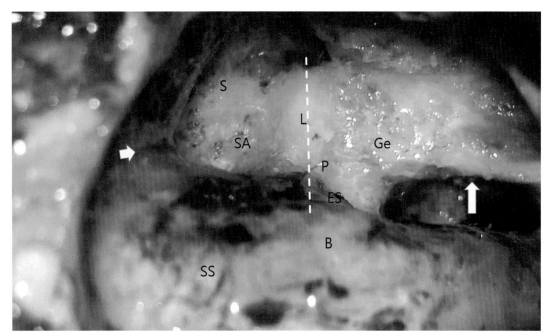

Figure 7-3. Microscopic view of complete mastoidectomy. Mastoid segment (arrow) and 2nd genu (Ge) of facial nerve identified. Contour of lateral (L), posterior (P), superior (S) semicircular canal and subarcuate artery (SA) are shown. Thinning of sigmoid sinus (SS) with Bony island of Bill's bar (B) and widening of sinudural angle (short arrow) were done with gentle drilling. Endolymphatic sac (ES) is located 60 degrees inside the point, where the Donaldson line (dotted line) meets the sigmoid sinus.

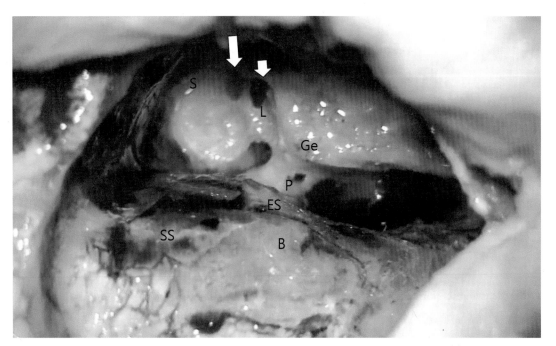

Figure 7-4. Microscopic view of during labyrinthectomy. Labyrinthectomy proceeds in the order of lateral (L) SCC, posterior SCC (P), and superior SCC (S). Because the ampulla of superior SCC (arrow) which is located superior to the ampulla of lateral SCC (short arrow) is a landmark to find the superior vestibular nerve and IAC, it should be preserved during labyrinthectomy.
Ge; 2nd genu of facial nerve, SS; sigmoid sinus, ES; endolymphatic sac, B; Bony island of Bill's bar

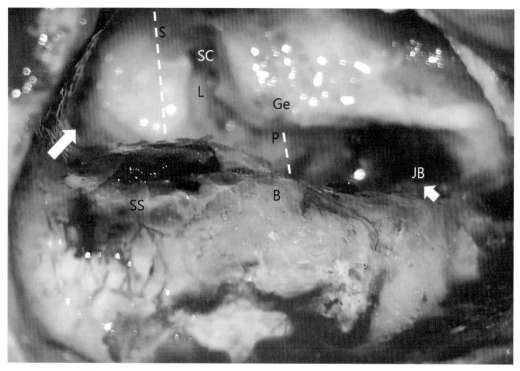

Figure 7-5. Microscopic view of post labyrinthectomy. The saccule is shown medial to lateral (L) canal Contour of ampullas of superior (S) and posterior (P) canal preserved for the landmarks of finding IAC (dotted line). When performing labyrinthectomy on a sclerotic mastoid, care should be taken as the narrow sinodural angle (arrow) and high jugular bulb (JB) (short arrow) may obscure the microscopic view.

6. troughing the IAC

Exposing only the outer small surface of the IAC can make surgery difficult with removing the tumor from IAC and additional drilling after dura incision of IAC causes iatrogenic damage of nerve. Therefore, make sure you have enough contours of about 270 degree of IAC before incision of dura of IAC, expose of the posterior fossa, and make the incision of dura parallel to IAC line (**Figure 7-6, 7**).

To define the IAC contour, troughing up and down the neighboring bony structure of IAC with drill. The boundary of drilling for the exposure were mastoid segment of facial canal anteriorly, dura of middle fossa superiorly, the posterior fossa and sigmoid sinus posteriorly, the jugular bulb inferiorly and the cochlear duct medially. Drilling is not recommended anterior and inferior to the cochlear aqueduct because this places cranial nerves IX, X and XI at risk.

7. Opening the IAC and Tumor removal

If possible, remove the bone component to expose the dura and perform the incision. For safe preservation of facial nerve, Identification of facial nerve with nerve stimulator both at the fundus and porus of canal are recommended. In particular, The Bill's bar divided the superior vestibular nerve laterally and a facial nerve medially at the fundus (**Figure 8**). The facial nerve in the middle of IAC could be moved or fanned by the mass, so care must be taken to remove the mass with monitoring system.

8. Fat obliteration and closure

The dural opening is packed with strips of fat stacked adjacent one to another, creating a dumbbell-shaped packing of fat through the dural defect. A watertight closure is required to prevent CSF leaks.

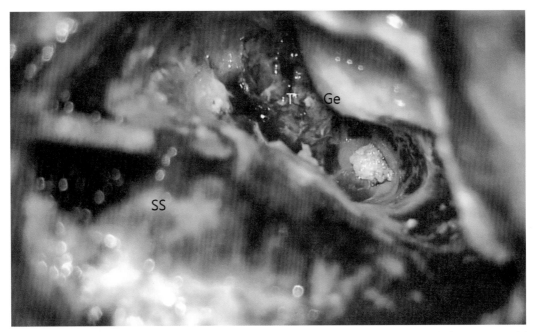

Figure 7-6. Tumor (T) is shown during the troughing the IAC. Enough drilling about 270 degree of IAC before incision of dura of IAC is recommended.
SS; sigmoid sinus, Ge; 2nd genu of facial nerve

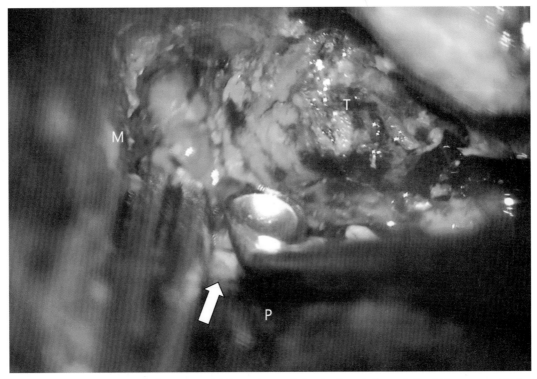

Figure 7-7. Bony portion around middle (M), posterior (P) fossa dura and sinodural angle (arrow) should be removed before incision of dura of IAC.

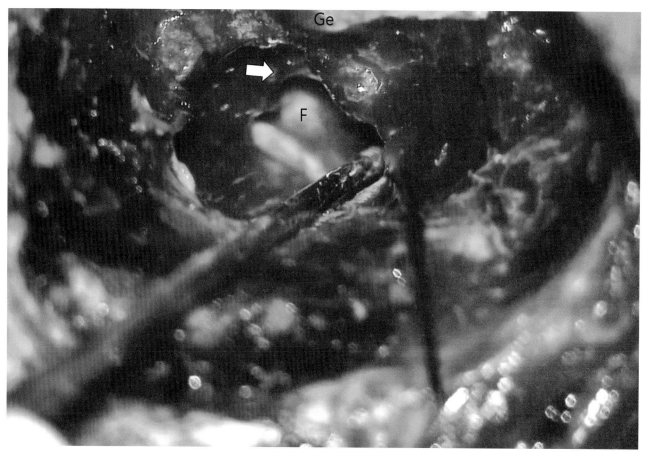

Figure 7-8. Microscopic view after tumor and vestibular nerve removal. Facial nerve (F) in the IAC runs medial to vertical crest (arrow) (Bill's bar) at the fundus of IAC.

III. Tip & Summary

1. Porus of IAC is located deeper than the fundus of IAC from the mastoid surface. Therefore, deep drilling from the mastoid cortex is required to expose the porus rather than the fundus of IAC.

2. In case of a high-riding jugular bulb, Press the dome gently with gelfoam to secure the field of view.

3. Superior and posterior canal ampullas are the reliable landmarks for finding IAC.

4. All bone superiorly and posteriorly to the medial middle and posterior fossa dura should be removed, if possible, prior to incision of dura of IAC

5. The facial nerve can be found with typically anatomy anterior to vertical crest (known as the Bill's bar) at the fundus.

6. In case of a medium sized tumor, facial nerve could be traced in the fundus of IAC proximally, porus of IAC distally and then remove the tumor without facial nerve trauma. In the case of a large tumor, Internal decompression volume reduction helps to avoid damaging the facial nerve and other neurovascular structures within the CPA by staying within the tumor capsule.

7. Be careful not to indirectly damage the facial nerve by stretching the tumor mass.

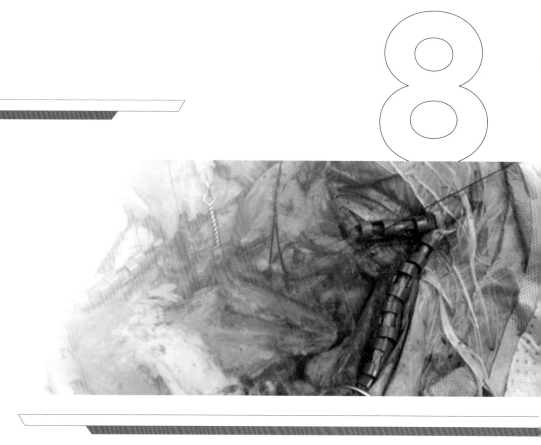

8

FAR LATERAL APPROACH

Je Beom Hong M.D., Han Kyu Kim M.D., Ph.D.

I. Introduction

The far lateral approach allows access to the dorsolateral compartment and ventromedial compartment of the posterior fossa. Through this approach, the cerebellomedullary and premedullary cistern, inferolateral and mid to lower clival area, ventral pons, and vertebrobasilar artery junction in the foramen magnum can be accessed with minimal brain retraction.

In 1972, Hammon first described the far lateral approach, and numerous modifications have been made since then.[5] With the addition of occipital condyle removal, jugular tubercle removal, and vertebral artery transposition, the area of application has gradually expanded. In 1986, Heors RC described a lateral foramen magnum approach.[6] He used condylar fossa re-

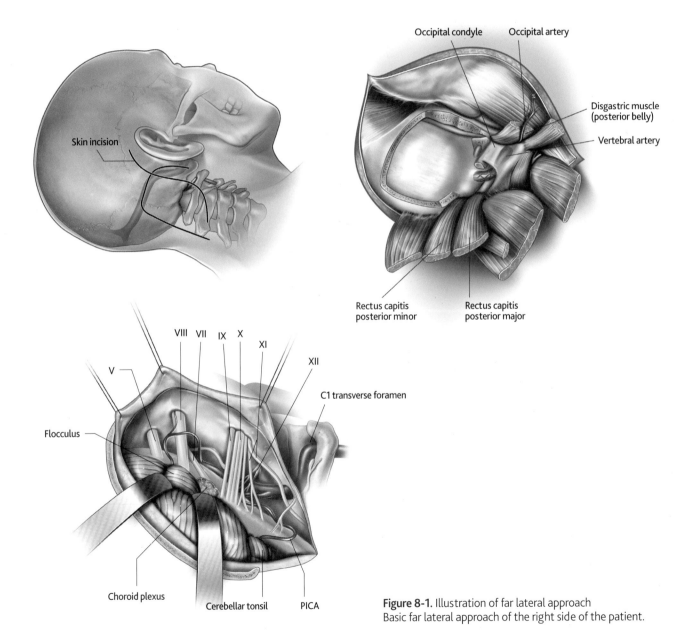

Figure 8-1. Illustration of far lateral approach
Basic far lateral approach of the right side of the patient.

moval and C1 hemilaminectomy. In 1986, in the same year, Perneczky A described jugular tubercle drilling while describing the posterolateral approach to the foramen magnum.[9] In 1991, Bertalanffy H and Seeger W described a transcondylar approach and vertebral artery transposition.[2] 1988 George described vertebral artery (VA) medial mobilization from C2 to its dural entrance point.[4] In 1994, Babu and Sekhar et al. reported medial reflection of the muscles including the sternocleidomastoid (SCM) muscle and medial transposition of the vertebral artery in an extreme lateral transcondylar approach.[1] A wider field of view could be obtained by performing the dural incision circumferentially around the vertebral artery.[11] extreme lateral infrajugular transcondylar-transtubercular exposure (ELITE) is a far lateral approach that includes posteroinferior mastoidectomy and jugular tubercle drilling.[8,10,12] Rhoton et al. systematized transcondylar, supracondylar, and paracondylar extensions of the far lateral approach.[13] In this article, we will describe the basic far lateral approach (**Figure 8-1**).

II. Procedure
(3 stages - muscular stage, extradural stage, intradural stage)

Basic far-lateral approach

It does not involve removal of the posterior part of the occipital condyle.
1) dissection of muscle along the posterolateral aspect of the craniocervical junction, C1 transverse process (TP) exposure
2) early identification of the vertebral artery (VA)
3) suboccipital craniotomy or craniectomy with C1 laminectomy

Then proceed with three variations

1) Transcondylar approach

- Through the occipital condyle, or atlanto-occipital joint and adjoining parts of the condyle.
- This approach allows more lateral access to the lower clivus and premedullary area.

2) Supracondylar approach

- Drilling above the occipital condyle.
- This approach allows access to the medial to the hypoglossal canal and jugular tubercle.

3) Paracondylar approach

- Drilling lateral to the occipital condyle (jugular process).
- This approach allows access to the posterior part of the jugular foramen, the posterior aspect of the facial nerve, and mastoid on the lateral side of the jugular foramen.

1. muscular stage (Figure 8-2)

1) Position

(1) Three quarter prone (Park bench) position
(2) The head is placed in a lateral position parallel to the floor and the upper shoulder is retracted anteroinferiorly.
(3) Lateral flexion of the head to allow natural retraction of the cerebellar tissue.
(4) The neck flexes so that the suboccipital triangle is widened.
(5) Allow the mastoid tip, inion, and spinous processes of the upper vertebrae to be palpable.

2) Skin incision

Horseshoe shaped scalp incision, inverted hockey stick incision or lazy "S" shaped scalp incision can be made.

3) Muscular dissection (2 stages)

(1) Nuchal
a. Sternocleidomastoid, trapezius - first layer, lateral reflection of the SCM exposes splenius capitis (**Figure 8-2a**).
b. Medial reflection of trapezius and splenius capitis exposes longissimus capitis.
c. When the longissimus capitis muscle is pushed down, the semispinalis capitis, superior oblique, inferior oblique muscle, and C1 TP emerge.

d. Medial displacement of the semispinalis muscle exposes the suboccipital triangle.

e. The suboccipital triangle is composed of the superior oblique, inferior oblique, and rectus capitis posterior major muscles, in which the vertebral artery and the C1 nerve are located.

f. Occipital artery (OA) emerges from the ECA posterior wall (at the mandible angle level), runs lateral to the IJV, parallel to the ECA, to the medial of the ECA, and runs posterolateral between the rectus capitis lateralis and the posterior belly of the digastric, then between the superior oblique and the posterior belly of the digastric. After that, when the occipital groove is present, it passes under the longissimus capitis muscle and when there is no occipital groove, it passes over the longissimus capitis muscle, then runs over the surface of the superior oblique muscle and over the semispinalis capitis muscle, passes through the attachment of the trapezius muscle and runs above the superior nuchal line do (**Figure 8-2b, 2c**).[3]

g. stylomastoid foramen
   - which transmits the facial nerve, is situated lateral to the jugular foramen (**Figure 8-2d**).

(2) Suboccipital (**Figure 8-2e**)
a. Suboccipital triangle
   - It is a triangle composed of obliquus capitis superior, obliquus capitis inferior, and rectus capitis posterior major muscle
   - a) third part of vertebral artery, b) dorsal ramus of nerve C1-suboccipital nerve, and c) suboccipital venous plexus exist inside

b. Depending on the lesion to be approached, the direction of retraction after dissection of the muscle may vary, but in most cases, the superior oblique is retracted laterally and rectus capitis major inferomedially.

c. V3 segment, C1 dorsal ramus, posterior arch of C1 in suboccipital triangle.

d. VA and C1 dorsal roots are buried in the vertebral venous plexus.

e. Occasionally, the posterior spinal artery and the posterior inferior cerebellar artery (PICA) originate from V3, so care must be taken not to misunderstand it as a muscular branch.

f. Also, there may be variations in the relationship between C1, C2, and VA. In some cases, there may be a bony defect, and there may be cases in which VA may appear at a location other than the C1 transverse foramen.

g. The rectus capitis lateralis is deeper than the superior oblique muscle and attaches to the jugular process at the posterior edge of the jugular tubercle. It starts at the upper surface of the transverse process of the atlas. attached to the lower surface of the jugular process. This muscle becomes an important landmark for the jugular foramen in the paracondylar approach.

h. The levator scapulae muscle lies below the C1 TP. The second segment of the vertebral artery lies medial to the levator scapulae muscle, and the carotid compartment of the parapharyngeal space is lateral.

i. Finally, dissection of the rectus capitis posterior minor muscle into the medial exposes the atlanto-occipital membrane.

j. vascular structures
   - The VA is deposited in the rich venous plexus, and when exposing or transposing the VA, it must be obliterated or partially removed.
   - The C1 nerve runs on the lower surface of the artery between the VA and the posterior arch of the atlas.
   - VA enters the vertebral canal from the lower part of the posterior atlanto-occipital membrane.
   - Muscular branches from VA can be divided if necessary during VA manipulation.
   - The posterior meningeal artery originates from the posterior surface of VA, but may also have intradural origin. At this time, it penetrates the arachnoid and supplies dura.

k. Osseous structures
   - In the C1 TP (transverse process), the rectus capitis lateralis muscle attaches to the anterior, and the superior oblique originates from the posterior portion of the upper surface. The inferior oblique attaches to the lateral tip. The levator scapulae, splenius cervicis, and scalene muscles attach to inferior and lateral surfaces of the TP.

Figure 8-2. Muscular stage of far lateral approach
From (a) to (e) shows the step by step exposure of the far lateral approach. (a) incision was made in a lazy S shaped fashion. (e) intraoperative picture of muscular stage using inverted hockey stick skin incision.

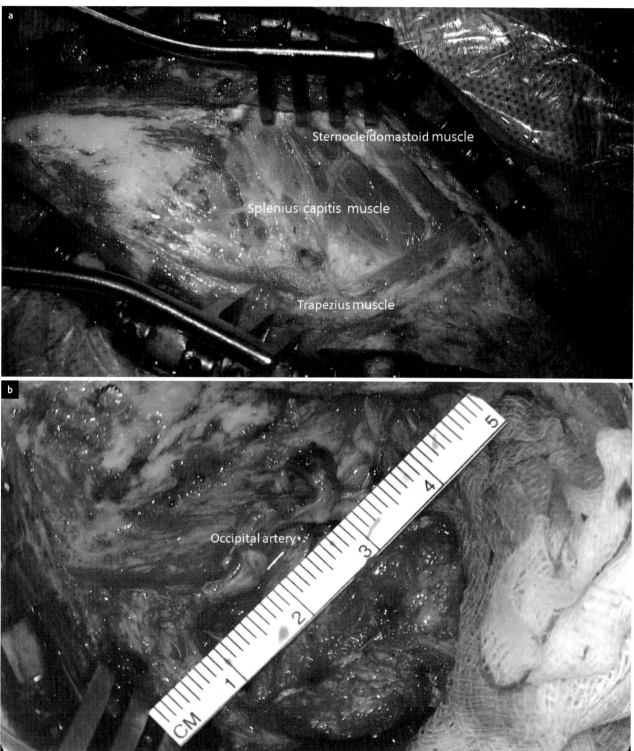

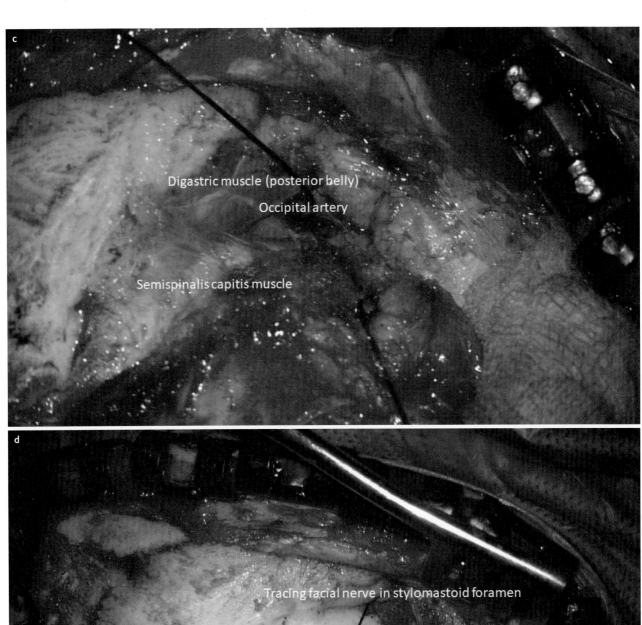

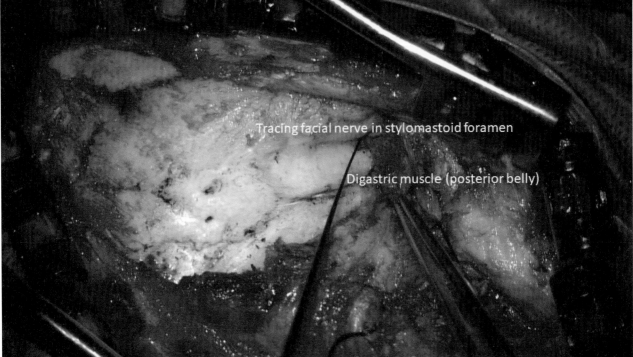

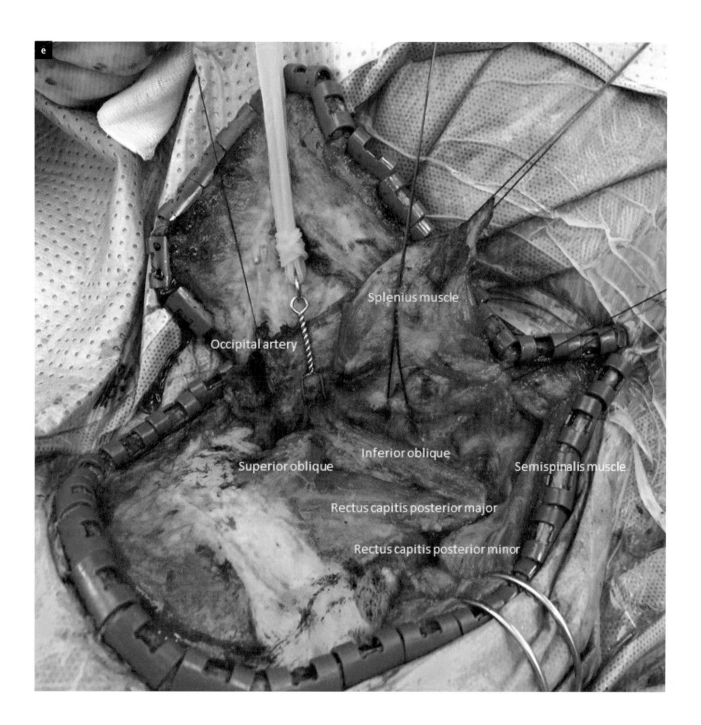

2. Extradural stage (Figure 8-3)

1) suboccipital craniotomy or craniectomy

- Exposing the occipital condyle.
- Remove more than half of the posterior arch of the atlas.
- VA mobilization can also be performed by removing the posterior root of the transverse foramen.
- The VA can be displaced medially to expose the atlanto-occipital joint.

(1) Important landmarks

a. Asterion - The site of the transition of the transverse sinus to the sigmoid sinus

b. Inion (external occipital protuberance) - 1 cm below the lower margin of the torcular herophili

c. Occipital condyles
- It projects downward along the lateral edge of the anterior half of the foramen magnum and articulates with the superior facet of the atlas.

d. Hypoglossal canal
- Pass 45 degrees in an anterolateral trajectory, positioned at a position of 10 o'clock, 2 o'clock in the foramen magnum. Therefore, when drilling the occipital condyle in the far lateral approach, the hypoglossal canal is first encountered in the medial aspect.
- The intracranial end is located 5 mm above the junction of the posterior and middle third of the occipital condyle, 5 mm below the jugular tubercle. The extracranial end of the hypoglossal canal is present in the junction of the anterior and middle third of the occipital condyle and medial to the jugular foramen. The average length of the condyle is 21 mm (range, 18-24 mm). The hypoglossal nerve, a meningeal branch of the ascending pharyngeal artery, and the venous plexus are present. The lateral aspect of the intracranial end of the hypoglossal canal is reached with removal of approximately the posterior third of the occipital condyle (8.4 mm of 21 mm). Laterally, the posterior 2/3 of the occipital condyle must be drilled for the hypoglossal canal to exist.

e. Jugular tubercle

- Above the hypoglossal canal, present in the medial to the lower half of the intracranial end of the jugular foramen
- CN IX, X, XI pass the posterior portion of the jugular tubercle. The jugular tubercle blocks the access to the basal cistern and the clivus anterior to the lower cranial nerves (LCN).

f. Jugular process
- If more lateral exposure is required, the jugular process is removed after detaching the rectus capitis lateralis muscle.

g. Condylar fossa
- Behind the occipital condyle is the condylar fossa, the posterior condylar emissary vein and the sigmoid sinus.

h. Jugular process
- It forms the posterior margin of the jugular foramen. The rectus capitis lateralis muscle attaches.

(2) Craniotomy

a. A basic lateral suboccipital craniotomy will be performed.
- It is bordered by superiorly transverse sinus, laterally sigmoid sinus and occipital condyle.

b. Laminectomy or laminotomy for the C1 posterior arch.
- The most important step at this time is to peel off the VA well.
- It is also important to dissociate the C2 spinal nerve root from the atlantoaxial joint.

c. VA manipulation
- Separate the VA from the transverse foramen by unroofing the foramen transversarium and displace it medial or lateral.
- The possible mutations in C1, C2, and VA should be carefully reviewed and proceeded with before surgery.

d. Then, transcondylar, supracondylar, and paracondylar extensions are performed.
- Transcondylar approach
  · Drill the posterior 1/3 of the condyle.
  · Meets the hypoglossal canal, which has a dark blue venous plexus wall.
  · If the lesion has not invaded the hypoglossal

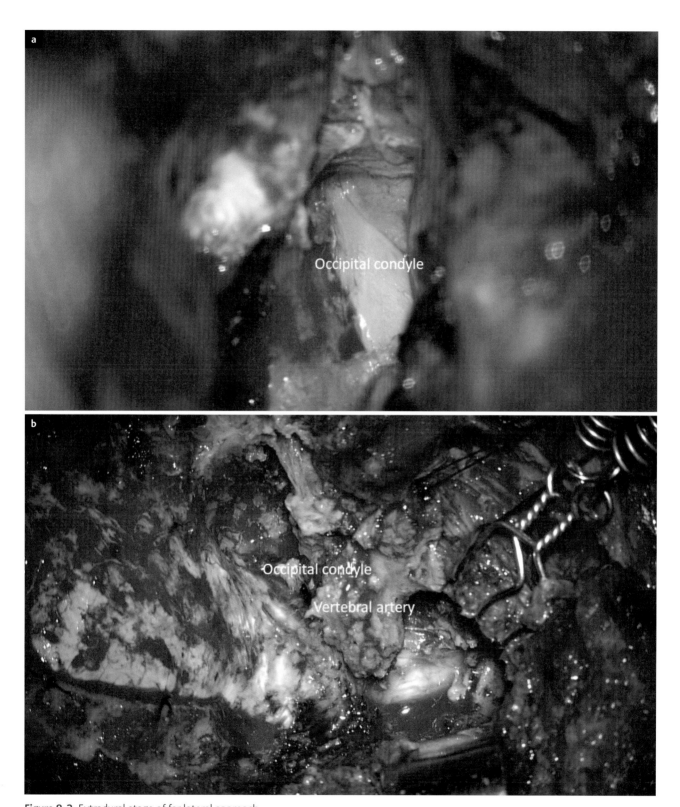

Figure 8-3. Extradural stage of far lateral approach
(a) intraoperative picture showing occipital condyle. (b) final picture of extradural stage of far lateral approach.

canal, the clivus can be accessed by performing condylectomy below and medial to the hypoglossal canal.

- Supracondylar extension
  · It is performed when access to the jugular foramen or upper medulla is required.
  · Removal of the posterior aspect of the jugular tubercle limited inferiorly by the hypoglossal canal, superiorly by the sigmoid sinus, laterally by the jugular bulb.
  · When drilling the jugular tubercle, be very careful with a diamond bur. This is because the spinal accessory nerve rootlets at the medial (dural) limit pass inward.
  · CN IX, X and XI pass through the neural compartment of the jugular foramen.
  · The supracondylar approach allows access to the petroclival junction and midclivus above the vagus nerve.
- Paracondylar approach
  · Can be used to access the jugular bulb, lower sigmoid sinus, meatal segment of the CN IX, X, XI.
  · The more lateral muscular flap, including the posterior belly of the digastric muscle, should be lifted.
  · Drilling should be done while paying attention to damage to CN IX, X, and XI through monitoring.
  · Perform drilling with the jugular process (an osseous protuberance at the posterior aspect of the jugular foramen).
  · Finally the lower part of the sigmoid sinus, the jugular bulb, jugular vein, the neural compartment of the jugular foramen, the pharyngeal segment of the internal carotid artery is exposed.

3. Intradural stage (Figure 8-4)

1) Dural opening
(1) The dural incision begins behind the sigmoid sinus and extends to the upper cervical area.(**Figure 8-4a**).
(2) Caution should be exercised for bleeding of the marginal sinus, the posterior meningeal artery (extradural origin or rarely intradural origin).

(3) Long midline incision and superior incision will be the basis. You can design it according to the lesion you want to access.
(4) Subsequently, cisterna magna incision can be performed to drain the cerebrospinal fluid to reduce cerebellar retraction.
(5) Exposed structures include the posterior spinal artery, dentate ligament, first cervical nerve, the spinal accessory nerve, and vertebral artery. The dentate ligament lies anteriorly between the vertebral artery and the ventral roots of C1 and posteriorly between the branches of the posterior spinal artery and spinal accessory nerve.
(6) The spinal accessory nerve originates in the spinal cord, ascends through the foramen magnum, and lies between the dentate ligament and dorsal root, posterior to the vertebral artery.
(7) The intradural vertebral artery lies anterior to the rootlets of the hypoglossal nerve and intersects with the basilar artery at the pontomedullary junction (**Figure 8-4b**).
(8) PICA emerges from the VA at the lower border of the pons, passes between the rootlets of CN IX, X, and XI, and runs to the lateral surface of the medulla.
(9) Structures those can cause bleeding are the transverse sinus, sigmoid sinus, marginal sinus, posterior meningeal artery (from intradural segment of the vertebral artery), posterior spinal artery (from VA at its dural cuff), meningeal branch of the ascending pharyngeal artery.
(10) Cranial nerves those can be accessed are CN V, VI, VII, VIII, IX, X, XI, XII (**Figure 8-4c~4h**).
(11) If the lesion extends to the cerebellopontine angle, it is better to extend the dural incision to the transverse-sigmoid sinus junction leaving a margin for safe closure.

2) Closure
(1) Close the dura as watertight as possible, and if the tension is too tight, close it using artificial dural material or allodermis.
(2) It is useful to leave and close the musculofascial cuff on the superior nuchal line.

Figure 8-4. Intradural stage of far lateral approach
(a) intraoperative picture after dura incision. (b~h) intraoperative pictures of structures those can be accessed via far lateral approach.

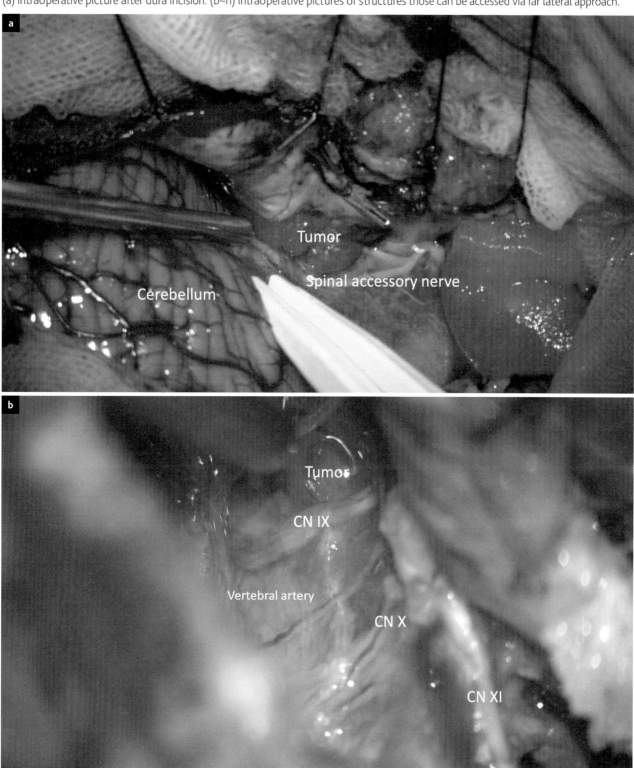

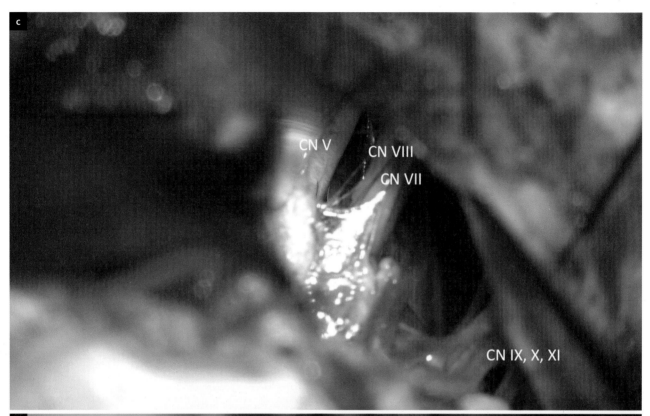

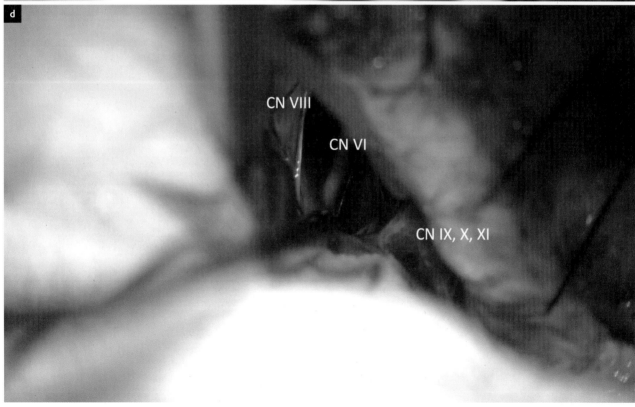

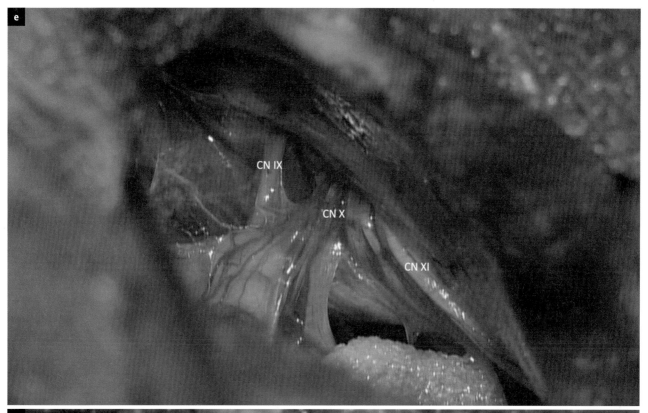

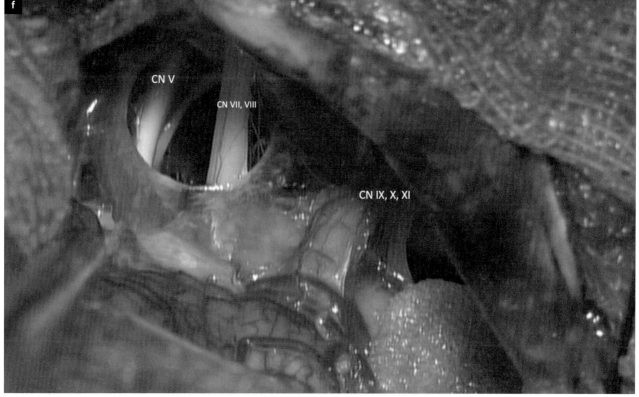

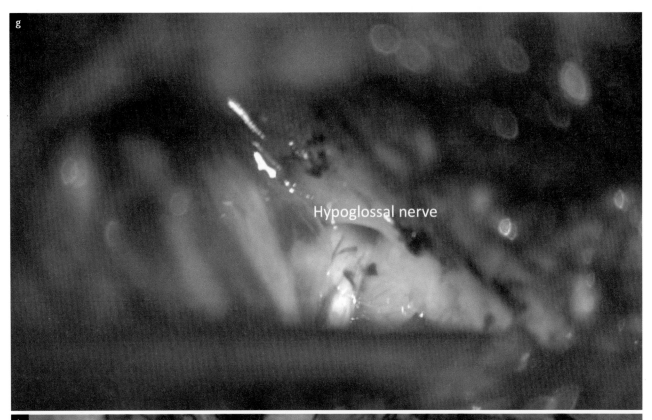

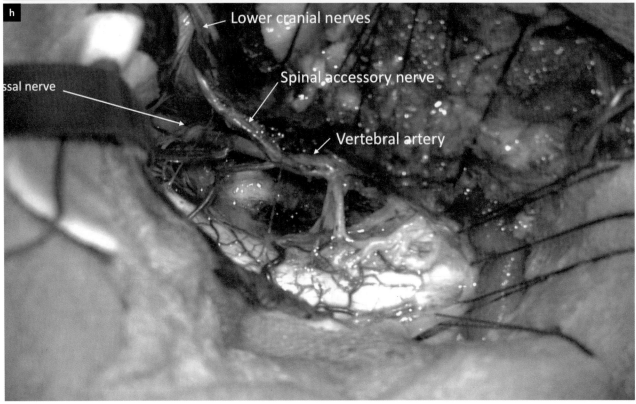

(3) Elevation of the muscles above the occipital squama in a single layer reduces flap dehiscence and allows the identification of important muscle landmarks - the suboccipital triangle, levator scapulae, and rectus capitis lateralis.

Anatomy to remember

Jugular foramen (3 compartments)

The superior of the jugular foramen is the petrous part of the temporal bone and the inferior is the occipital bone.

(1) Sigmoid compartment
  - sigmoid sinus, the jugular bulb, the meningeal branches of the ascending pharyngeal, vertebral, or occipital arteries exist
  - dural fold - the presence of a dural fold between the superior intrajugular process in the middle of the jugular foramen and the inferior intrajugular process in the jugular tubercle, dividing the sigmoid and neural compartments
(2) Neural compartment (Intermediate portion)
  - The accessory (CN XI), vagus (CN X), and glossopharyngeal (CN IX) nerves are present.
  - It is divided into glossopharyngeal meatus (anterior) and the vagal meatus (posterior) by the dural septum.
  - glossopharyngeal meatus
    the glossopharyngeal nerve, its tympanic branch (Jacobson's nerve)
  - vagal meatus
    vagus nerve, its auricular branch (Arnold's nerve), accessory nerve
(3) Petrous compartment
  - Between neural compartment and petroclival synchondrosis, passing inferior petrosal sinus

Occipital bone (3 part - squamous part, basilar part, condylar part)

(1) squamous part
  - external occipital protuberance (inion)
    · torcula lower margin 1 cm superior to the inion
  - superior nuchal line

  · sternocleidomastoid, trapezius, splenius capitis, semispinalis capitis tendinous insertion
  - the asterion (a confluence of the lambdoid, parietomastoid, occipitomastoid sutures)
    · Transverse sinus transition to sigmoid sinus
  - digastric groove (area where the digastric muscle posterior belly attaches)
    · It is also a landmark of the sigmoid sinus or the landmark of the facial nerve coming out of the stylomastoid foramen.
  - inferior nuchal line
    · Area of attachment of suboccipital muscles (superior oblique, rectus capitis posterior major, rectus capitis posterior minor)
(2) condylar part (Consists of occipital condyle, condylar fossa, and jugular tubercle)
  - condylar fossa
    · The posterior condylar emissary vein (connected to the sigmoid sinus) emerges.
  - occipital condyle
    · Forms the superior articular facet of the atlas and articulate, atlanto-occipital joint
  - The jugular tubercle
    · It is located between the hypoglossal canal and the jugular bulb and forms the roof of the hypoglossal canal and the floor of the jugular foramen.
    · It can also be divided into two compartments.
    a. condylar compartment
      - below the hypoglossal canal
      - Drilling here accesses the lower clivus.
    b. jugular tubercle compartment
      - above the hypoglossal canal
      - Drilling here accesses the jugular foramen, lateral and anterior medullary spaces.
(3) basilar part
  a thick, somewhat quadrilateral piece in front of the foramen magnum and directed towards the pharynx

III. Illustrative case (Figure 8-5~7)

A 68-year-old male visited our hospital with complaints of gait disturbance and decreased limb muscle strength. The imaging study showed foramen magnum meningioma ranging from the lower clivus to the upper C1 level (**Figure 8-5**). The brainstem was severely compressed. Surgical removal was planned and it was decided to be removed through a far lateral approach. The patient's body was placed in a park bench position and the head was placed parallel to the floor. Curvilinear lazy S shaped skin incision was made, and muscle dissection was performed with coagulation and cut of the occipital artery. After that, suboccipital craniotomy and C1 laminectomy were performed. After dural incision, the tumor was exposed, and the tumor was removed while preserving the lower cranial nerve (**Figure 8-6**). When it was judged that the tumor was sufficiently removed, duroplasty was performed using artificial dura, and the bone flap and muscle were fixed in their original positions and the operation was completed. The postoperative magnetic resonance imaging (MRI) showed sufficiently removed tumor (**Figure 8-7**). The patient complained of temporary dysphagia, but improved after rehabilitation and was discharged.

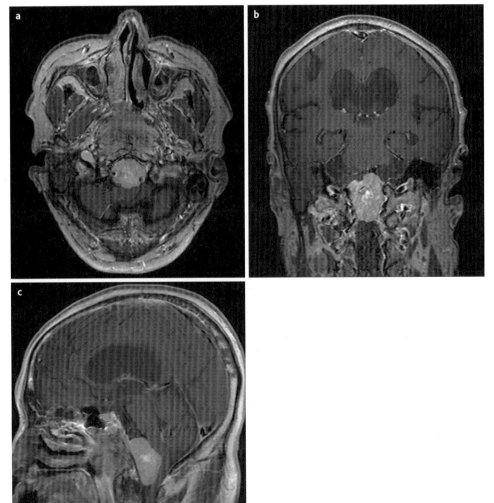

Figure 8-5. Preoperative magnetic resonance imaging (MRI) of illustrative case T1 enhanced axial (a), coronal (b), sagittal (c) MRI.

Figure 8-6. Intraoperative pictures of illustrative case
Tumor was dissected from lower cranial nerves and vertebral artery. The pictures before (a) and after (b) the tumor removal

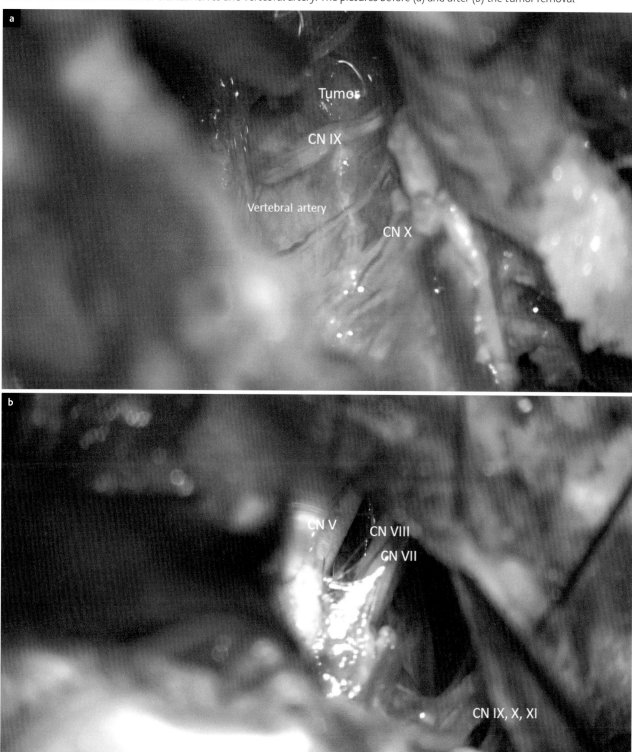

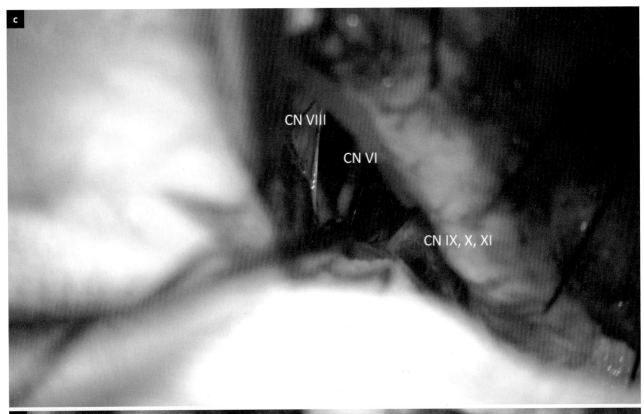

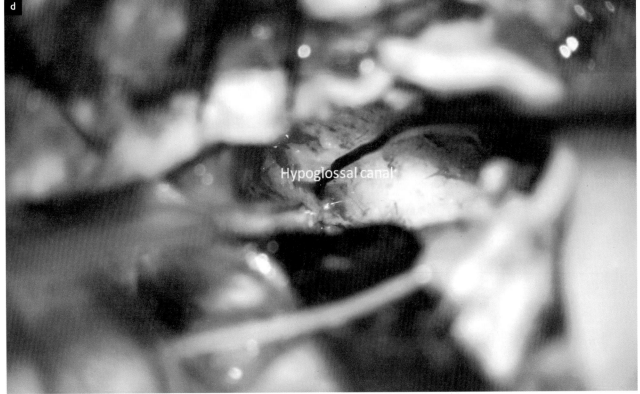

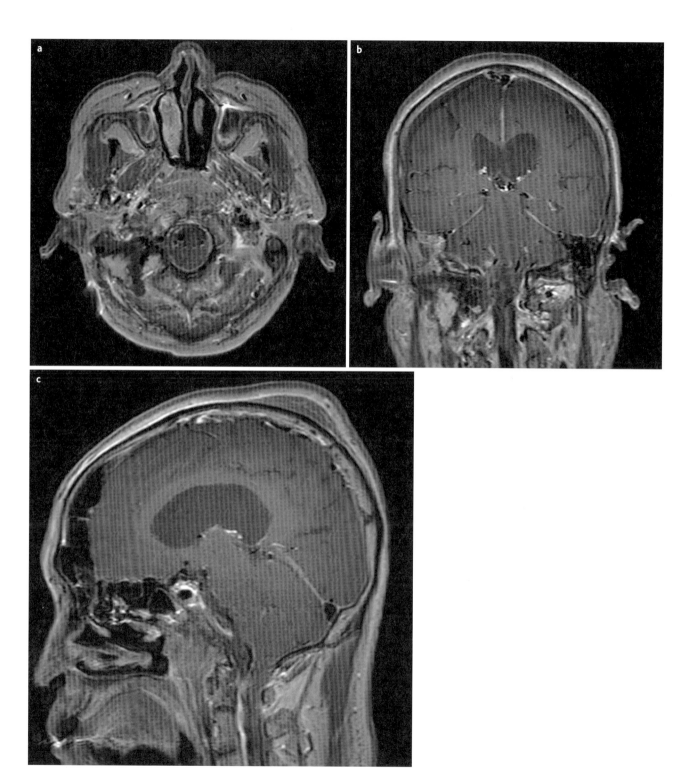

Figure 8-7. Postoperative MRI of illustrative case
T1 enhanced axial (a), coronal (b), sagittal (c) MRI.

IV. Surgical tip & pitfall

1. Even touching the nerves can cause dysfunction, so it is best not to touch the nerves as much as possible. Since LCNs travel to the posterior of the VA, the risk of LCN damage can be reduced if the tumor is approached from the anterior side of the VA. VA runs anterior to the rootlets of lower cranial nerves.

2. Be careful as there are cases where PICA originates in the extracranial space (20%).

3. The posterior spinal artery should also be taken into consideration, as the origin may come from intra-dural VA, extradural VA or PICA.

4. There may be variations in VA course and atlanto-occipital junction, so it is important to carefully examine the CT angiography before surgery (ex., ponticulus posticus).[7]

5. It has been reported that partial drilling of the posterior occipital condyle is safe for instability (33-75% of the condyle). However, the possibility of instability should be kept in mind.

6. If the brainstem is severely compressed due to a tumor within the foramen magnum, the neck flexion should not be excessive and motor evoked potential and somatosensory evoked potential should be checked after the position.

7. The dura should be closed as watertight as possible, and it is important to close redundantly without tension even with dural substitutes if necessary.

REFERENCES

1. Babu RP, Sekhar LN, Wright DC. Extreme lateral transcondylar approach: technical improvements and lessons learned. J Neurosurg 1994;81(1):49-59.

2. Bertalanffy H, Seeger W. The dorsolateral, suboccipital, transcondylar approach to the lower clivus and anterior portion of the craniocervical junction. Neurosurgery 1991;29(6):815-21.

3. Di G, Fang X, Hu Q, Zhou W, Jiang X. A microanatomical study of the far lateral approach. World Neurosurg 2019;127:e932-42.

4. George B, Dematons C, Cophignon J. Lateral approach to the anterior portion of the foramen magnum. Application to surgical removal of 14 benign tumors: technical note. Surg Neurol 1988;29(6):484-90.

5. Hammon WM, Kempe LG. The posterior fossa approach to aneurysms of the vertebral and basilar arteries. J Neurosurg 1972;37(3):339-47.

6. Heros RC. Lateral suboccipital approach for vertebral and vertebrobasilar artery lesions. J Neurosurg 1986;64(4):559-62.

7. Li T, Yin Y-H, Qiao G-Y, Wang H-W, Yu X-G. Three-dimensional evaluation and classification of the anatomy variations of vertebral artery at the craniovertebral junction in 120 patients of basilar invagination and atlas occipitalization. Oper Neurosurg (Hagerstown) 2019;17(6):594-602.

8. Mintelis A, Sameshima T, Bulsara KR, Gray L, Friedman AH, Fukushima T. Jugular tubercle: Morphometric analysis and surgical significance. J Neurosurg 2006;105(5):753-7.

9. Perneczky A. The Posterolateral Approach to the Foramen Magnum. Berlin, Heidelberg: Springer;1986.pp460-6.

10. Rennert RC, Hoshide R, Brandel MG, Steinberg JA, Martin JR, Meltzer HS, et al. Surgical relevance of pediatric skull base maturation for the far-lateral and extreme-lateral infrajugular transcondylar-transtubercular exposure approaches. J Neurosurg Pediatr 2019;24(1):85-91.

11. Salas E, Sekhar LN, Ziyal IM, Caputy AJ, Wright DC. Variations of the extreme-lateral craniocervical approach: anatomical study and clinical analysis of 69 patients. J Neurosurg Spine 1999;90(1):206-19.

12. Wanibuchi M, Fukushima T, Zenga F, Friedman AH. Simple identification of the third segment of the extracranial vertebral artery by extreme lateral inferior transcondylar-transtubercular exposure (ELITE). Acta Neurochir (Wien) 2009;151(11):1499-503.

13. Wen HT, Rhoton AL Jr, Katsuta T, de Oliveira E. Microsurgical anatomy of the transcondylar, supracondylar, and paracondylar extensions of the far-lateral approach. J Neurosurg 1997;87(4):555-85.

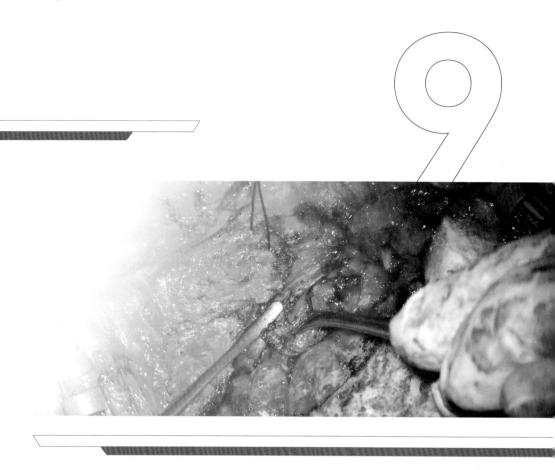

9

TRANSJUGULAR APPROACH:

FAR-LATERAL APPROACHES FOR THE MANAGEMENT OF POSTERIOR FOSSA TUMORS WITH JUGULAR FORAMEN EXTENSION

Ho Jun Seol M.D., Ph.D., Won Jae Lee M.D., Kwan Park M.D., Ph.D.

I. Introduction

The jugular foramen (JF) is formed by the petrous part of temporal bone anteriorly and the occipital bone posteriorly (**Figure 9-1a**).[1,2] The structures passes the JF included the glossopharyngeal nerve (cranial nerve [CN] IX), vagus nerve (CN X), accessory nerve (CN XI), sigmoid sinus (SS), jugular bulb (JB), inferior petrosal sinus (IPS), and meningeal branches of the ascending pharyngeal and occipital artery (**Figure 9-1b**).[3,4]

The complexity of the JF requires exquisite surgical anatomy knowledge to access this region. According to the natures and extents of the disease, several op-

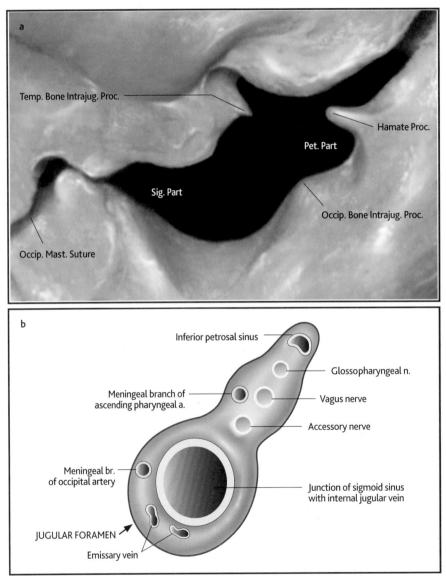

Figure 9-1. (a) The osseous relationships of the jugular foramen (JF). The large posterolateral sigmoid part and the small anteromedial petrosal part is divided by the fibrous intrajugular septum which connects the intrajugular process of temporal bone and the intrajugular process of occipital bone. (b) The schematic drawing of traversing structures of the JF.

erative approaches had been introduced to access the JF and adjacent areas. The posterior approach directed through the posterior fossa is one of the most familiar approach to the neurosurgeon.[5] Generally, intradural pathologies that extends into the JF can be accessed by the retrosigmoid (RS) approach and the far-lateral approach which is an extended modification of the RS approach. The jugular process (JP) of the occipital bone, which forms the posterior margin of the JF is a key anatomical structure of the far-lateral approach to the JF (**Figure 9-2**).[6,7] The JP of occipital bone can

be localized by identifying the rectus capitis lateralis muscle (RCLM) that connects the transverse process (TP) of atlas with the JP of the occipital bone (**Figure 9-3a**). Drilling of the JP of the occipital bone in the paracondylar location (which is called 'paracondylar extension of far-lateral approach') allow us to access the posterior margin of the jugular bulb (**Figure 9-3b, 3c**).[8] According to the extent of disease, transcondylar, supracondylar and several modifications of these approaches can be applied during far-lateral approach for the JF.

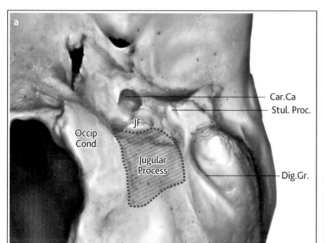
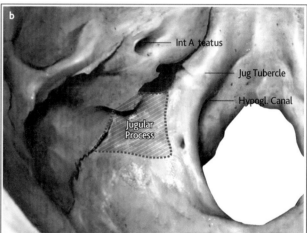

Figure 9-2. The artistic illustrations of the jugular foramen (JF) and the jugular process (JP) of occipital bone, inferior (a) and superior (b) views. JP of the occipital bone forms the posterior edge of JF. This is a bony landmark to access the JF during the far-lateral approach.

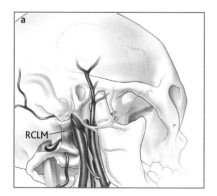
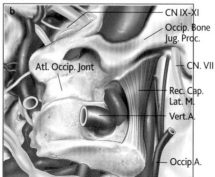
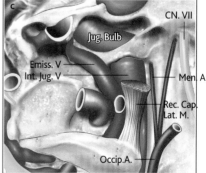

Figure 9-3. The artistic illustrations showing the rectus capitis lateralis muscle (RCML) and adjacent neurovascular structures. (a) The RCML arises from the superior surface of the transverse process of the atlas (C1) and inserts to the inferior surface of the jugular process (JP) of the occipital bone. The jugular bulb can be exposed after the removal of the RCML and JP of the occipital bone (b and c).

During the skull base surgery, comprehensive understanding of bony anatomy and its' relationship with adjacent neurovascular structures is imperative. Preoperative thin-section computed tomography (CT) with contrast-enhancement is helpful in figuring out the relationship of skull base and vascular structures such as sigmoid sinus, emissary veins, vertebral artery (VA), other intracranial arteries of posterior circulation, and venous plexus around the cranio-cervical junction. It also useful in identifying the intraosseous course of foramina which the CNs passing through. Intraoperative use of CT scan using navigation system increase the accuracy of meticulous drilling of skull base. In addition, Proton Density (PD) weighted magnetic resonance imaging (MRI) sequence is beneficial in evaluating the courses of CNs. Prior to surgery, knowing the spatial relationship between the tumor and the CNs at risk is important in surgical planning.

In this chapter, we present stepwise surgical illustration of transcondylar, supracondylar and paracondylar approaches of far-lateral approach for accessing the JF.

II. Procedures

1. Illustrative case

The MR images from a 41 year-old female patient presenting with a headache and dysphagia showing a left sided large cerebellopontine angle meningioma (**Figure 9-4**). The internal auditory canal, sigmoid sinus and the jugular bulb were invaded by the tumor. The tumor also extended into the carotid space through the jugular foramen and the hypoglossal canal (HC). The patient underwent surgical resection of the tumor through the far-lateral approach and its' transconylar, supracondylar and paracondylar extension.

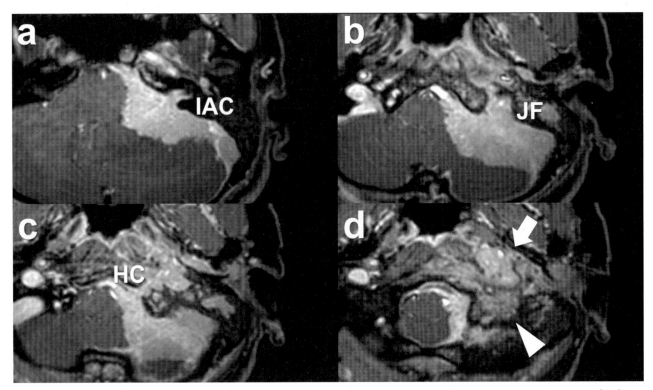

Figure 9-4. (a, b, and c) The MR images showing cerebello-pontine angle meningioma invading the internal auditory canal (IAC), the jugular foramen (JF), and the hypoglossal canal (HC). (d) The tumor extended into the carotid space (white arrow) through the JF and HC. The base of occipital bone was also involved by the tumor (white arrow head).

2. Patient's position and skin incision

A modified park-bench position was used (**Figure 9-5a**). Ipsilateral shoulder taped down and the patient's body should be secured to the operating table. This position allows the full range of tilting of the operating table. The patient's trunk is elevated about 15-20 degree to maintain venous return. The head is rotated downward slightly, and the mastoid bone is the highest point. The head slightly turned down to the floor, hence the angle between the shoulder and neck is widened. The inverted U shape skin incision was designed (**Figure 9-5b**). The incision started at the level of TP of atlas and curved at the level of pinna and downed to the Inion until the level of C3.

3. Exposure the suboccipital triangle.

After the dissection of individual neck muscle, suboccipital triangle consisted with the superior oblique capitis muscle (SOCM), the inferior oblique capitis muscle (IOCM), and the rectus capitis posterior major muscle (RCP Maj.) was exposed (**Figure 9-6**). VA within the vertebral venous plexus and fat tissue can be found within the suboccipital triangle.

The origins and insertions of the posterior neck muscles during the far-lateral approach were described in **table 9-1**.

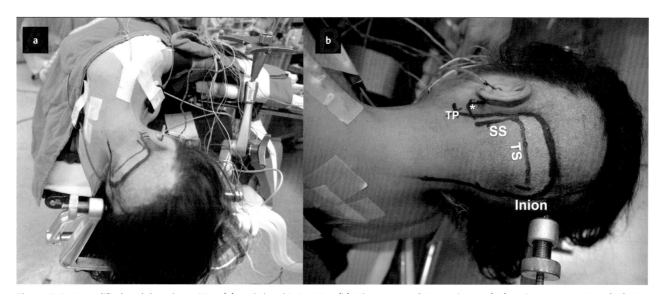

Figure 9-5. A modified park bench position (a) and the skin incision (b). The course of sigmoid sinus (SS) and transverse sinus (TS), the transverse process (TP) of atlas (C1), and the tip of mastoid process (asterisk) were marked. The incision started at the level of TP of C1 and curved at the level of pinna and downed to the Inion until the level of C3.

Table 9-1. Origins and insertions of posterior neck muscles

Muscles	Origin	Insertion
SOCM	TP of C1	Inferior nuchal line
IOCM	SP of C2	TP of C1
RCP Maj. m.	SP of C2	Inferior nuchal line
RCP Min. m.	Posteior arch of C1	Inferior nuchal line

SOCM: superior oblique capitis muscle, IOCM: inferior oblique capitis muscle, RCP Maj.: rectus capitis posterior major, RCP Min.: rectus capitis posterior minor, TP: transverse process, SP: spinous process

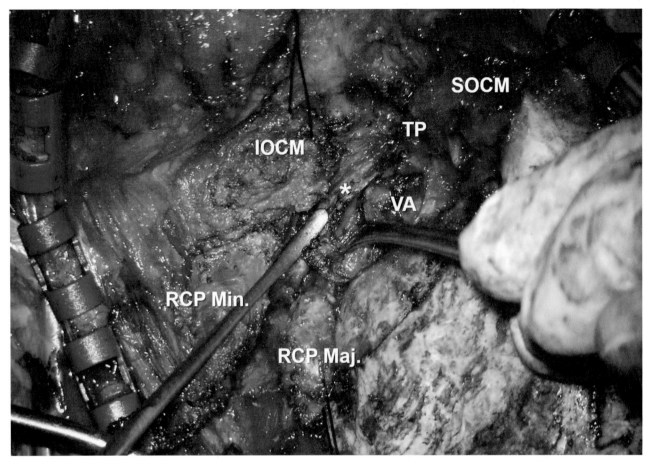

Figure 9-6. The muscles consisting the suboccipital triangle were dissected and reflected. transverse process (TP) of C1 is a bony landmark for identifying the inferior oblique capitis muscle (IOCM) and superior oblique capitis muscle (SOCM). The posterior arch of C1 (asterisk) and the vertebral artery (VA) were identified.
RCP Maj.: rectus capitis posterior major muscle, RCP Min: rectus capitis posterior minor muscle.

4. Paracondylar approach

After the resection of posterior arch of the atlas (C1), posterior wall of neural foramen of the C1 was unroofed and the VA was transposed downward using vessel loop. The RCLM originated at the TP of C1 and inserted to the JP of occipital bone was identified

(Figure 9-7a). After detachment of the RCML from JP of occipital bone, JP of occipital bone which forming the posterior edge of JF was drilled out to expose the jugular bulb (Figure 9-7b).

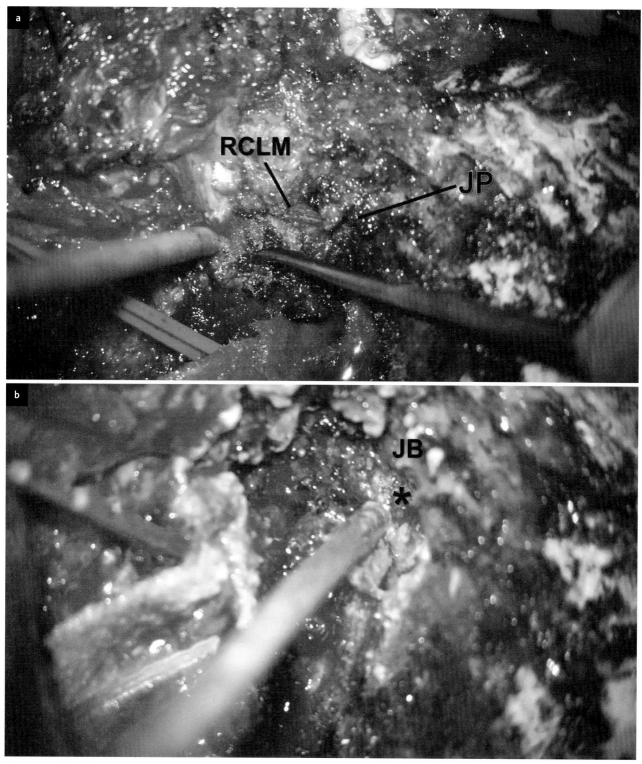

Figure 9-7. (a) In this case, the rectus capitis lateralis muscle (RCML) was invaded by the tumor. The vertebral artery was transposed inferiorly using vessel loop. (b) After drilling of the jugular process (JP) of occipital bone, the jugular bulb (JB) (asterisk) was identified. The JB was obstructed due to tumor invasion.

5. Transcondylar and supracondylar approach

After suboccipital craniotomy, posterior fossa dura was exposed (**Figure 9-8a**). The occipital condyle (OC) was identified, and posterior third of the OC was drilled until the HC was exposed (Transcondylar approach). Direct nerve stimulator is helpful to identify the course of hypoglossal nerve in the HC. After identifying the HC, drilling of the OC above the HC allows the extradural removal of the jugular tubercle the part of occipital bone located superior to the HC (**Figure 9-8b**). A surgical view after the completion of bone work for the far-lateral transcondylar, supracondylar and paracondylar approaches (**Figure 9-8c**).

6. Postoperative view and images

Tumor was removed, and the final surgical view showed the course of lower cranial nerves entering to the JF (**Figure 9-9**). Postoperative CT scans showed the result of bone work after the far-lateral approach (**Figure 9-10**). Posterior half of neural foramen of atlas was unroofed to transpose the VA. JP of occipital bone, OC, and jugular tubercle were drilled, and anterior two-thirds of OC was left.

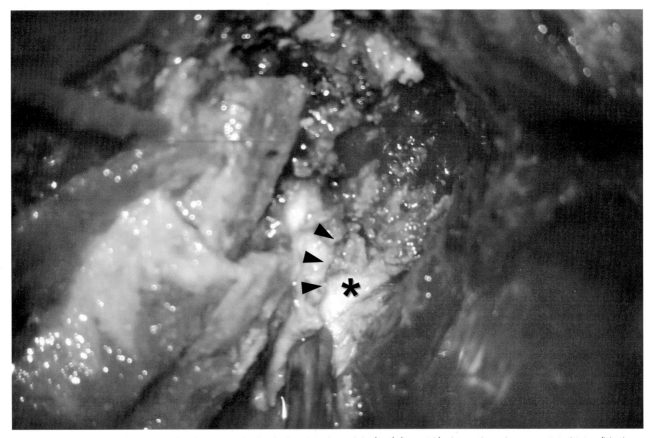

Figure 9-8a. Transcondylar approach. The posterior third of occipital condyle (OC) (asterisk) above the atlanto-occipital joint (black arrow heads) was identified and drilled out to access the lower clivus and in front of the medulla.

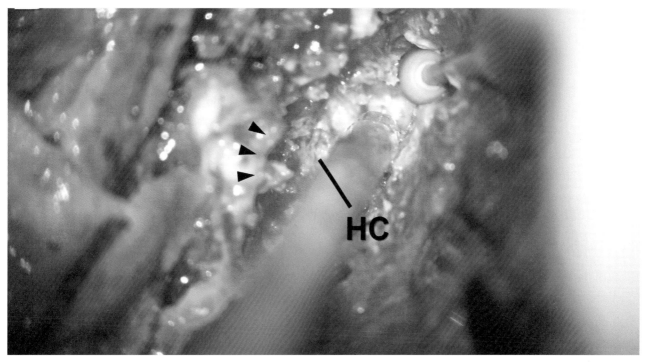

Figure 9-8b. Supracondylar approach. Drilling of the OC above the hypoglossal canal (HC) allows extradural removal of the jugular tubercle. This provides the wider surgical space in front of the brain stem.

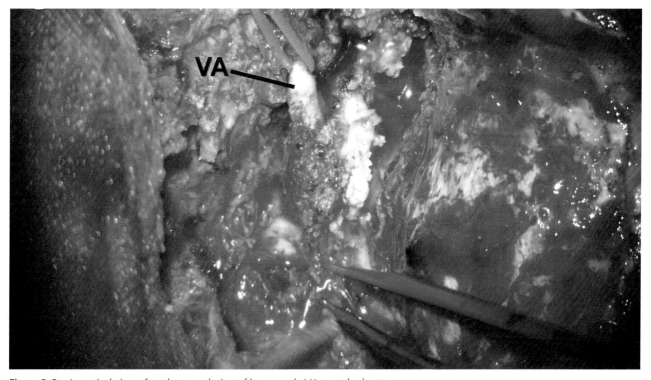

Figure 9-8c. A surgical view after the completion of bone work. VA: vertebral artery.

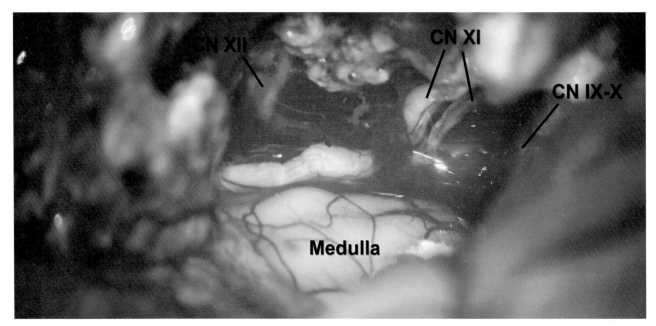

Figure 9-9. Final surgical view showing the course of lower cranial nerves after tumor resection CN (cranial nerve).

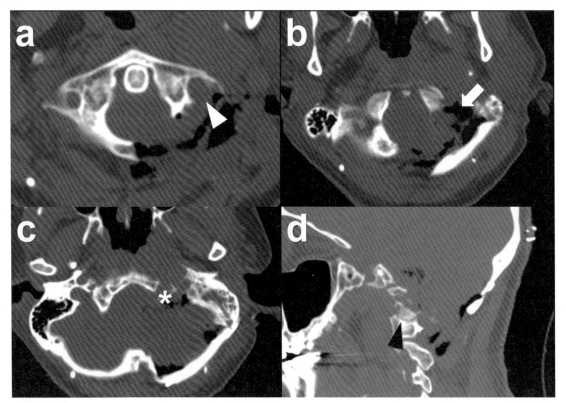

Figure 9-10. Postoperative CT images after far-lateral transcondylar, supracondylar, and paracondylar approach.
(a) Posterior half of the neural foramen of C1 (white arrow head) was unroofed to transpose the VA. (b, c) The jugular process of occipital bone (white arrow) and jugular tubercle (asterisk) were drilled. (d) Anterior two-thirds of atlanto-occipital joint was preserved (black arrow head).

III. Tip and summary

Muscular stage

During the muscular stage, important anatomical land marks are the TP and the posterior arch of the C1. Complete skeletonization of the VA is not necessary. The VA can be stay within the vertebral venous plexus and fat tissue. Manual palpation using finger and checking the arterial flow using Doppler ultrasound are useful method to identify the location of VA during the dissection.

Bony stage

Identification of the groove for VA of C1 is important step to detach the VA from the C1. The horizontal portion of V3 segment of VA should be mobilized and protected to avoid the VA injury. Then, posterior arch of C1 can be drilled safely.

During the paracondylar approach, TP of C1 is an important landmark for identifying the RCML. JP of occipital bone can be reached by following the course of RCML.

Emissary vein from the vertebral venous plexus to the sigmoid sinus often pass the base of the occipital bone. It can be handled safely after circumferential drilling of the bone around the emissary vein (**Figure 9-11**).

Smooth and safe drilling of the posterior thirds of OC until exposure of hard bone covering the HC is imperative to prevent CN XII injury. Identification of the HC is a first step to perform the transcondylar and supracondylar approach. Preoperative preparation of neurophysiologic monitoring for lower cranial nerves and the use of direct nerve stimulator are helpful.

Figure 9-11. Intraoperative photos showing the handling of an emissary vein. The vein passed the base of occipital bone, and drains the venous blood from vertebral venous plexus to the sigmoid sinus. Circumferential drilling of the occipital bone was performed (a). After coagulation of the vein (b), it can be amputated safely (c).

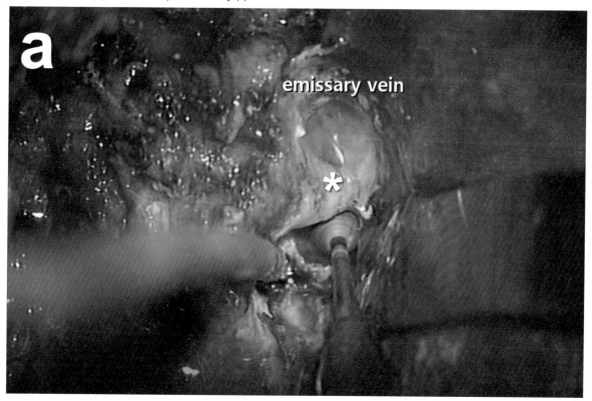

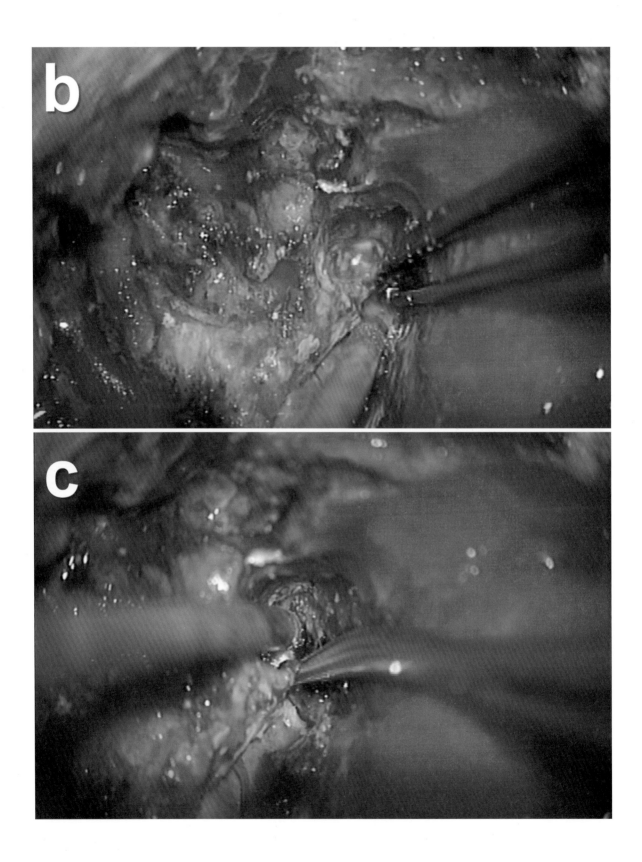

REFERENCE

1. Singh O and J MD. Anatomy, Head and Neck, Jugular Foramen StatPearls Treasure Island (FL); 2021.

2. Bernard F, Zemmoura I, Cottier JP, Fournier HD, Terrier LM and Velut S. The interperiosteodural concept applied to the jugular foramen and its compartmentalization. J Neurosurg 2018;129:770-8.

3. Rhoton AL, Jr. and Buza R. Microsurgical anatomy of the jugular foramen. J Neurosurg 1975;42:541-50.

4. Bond JD and Zhang M. Compartmental Subdivisions of the Jugular Foramen: A Review of the Current Models. World Neurosurg 2020;136:49-57.

5. Katsuta T, Rhoton AL, Jr. and Matsushima T. The jugular foramen: microsurgical anatomy and operative approaches. Neurosurgery 1997;41:149-201; discussion 201-2.

6. Ma SC, Liu S, Agazzi S and Jia W. The Jugular Process: A Key Anatomical Landmark for Approaches to the Jugular Foramen. World Neurosurg 2020;135:e686-e694.

7. Komune N, Matsuo S, Miki K, Matsushima K, Akagi Y, Kurogi R, Iihara K, Matsushima T, Inoue T and Nakagawa T. Microsurgical Anatomy of the Jugular Process as an Anatomical Landmark to Access the Jugular Foramen: A Cadaveric and Radiological Study. Oper Neurosurg (Hagerstown) 2019;16:486-95.

8. Wen HT, Rhoton AL, Jr., Katsuta T and de Oliveira E. Microsurgical anatomy of the transcondylar, supracondylar, and paracondylar extensions of the far-lateral approach. J Neurosurg 1997;87:555-85.

Video 9-1. An operation video of the illustrative case.

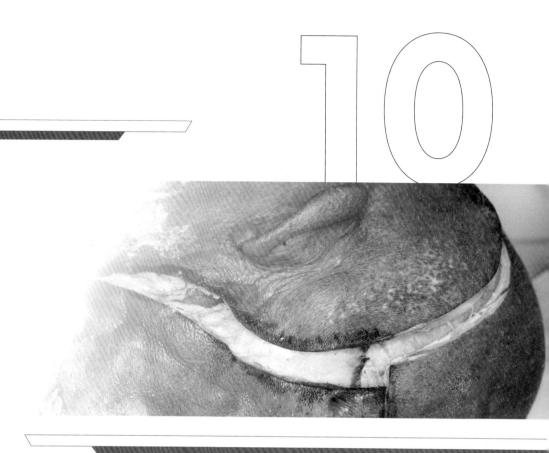

10

ANTEROLATERAL APPROACH TO CRANIOCERVICAL JUNCTION

Hun Ho Park M.D., Ph.D., Kyu Sung Lee M.D., Ph.D.
Sébastien Froelich M.D., Bernard George M.D.

I. Introduction

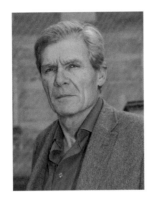

The anterolateral approach is a skull base approach to the craniocervical junction (CCJ) developed by Bernard George more than a decade ago, but still unfamiliar among skull base surgeons. Herein, the surgical technique of anterolateral approach is described step-by-step with its indications and limitations to CCJ.

The V2 segment of the vertebral artery (VA) can be exposed through an anterolateral approach, passing medially to the sternocleidomastoid muscle and laterally to the internal jugular vein. The safest method to expose the V2 segment of VA is to first reach the transverse process of C1 by retracting the longus colli muscle. Then, cutting the digastric, rectus capitis lateralis, superior and inferior oblique, and levator scapulae muscles from their attachments to the transverse process of C1 permit access to the prevertebral space. The V2 segment of VA can also be freed by opening the transverse process along the subperiosteal plane.

The approach provides access to the prevertebral space and it is very efficient for extra- and intra-dural tumors located anterolateral to CCJ with extension anywhere from C0 to C7 including the occipital condyle, atlanto-occipital joint, lateral mass and anterior arch of C1, odontoid process, and the body of C2. The limits of the approach are the jugular foramen, superiorly and the contralateral VA, medially. The approach can also be combined with other skull base approaches and modified according to the extent of lesion.

The anterolateral approach is one of the best approaches for resecting ventrally located lesions with lateral extension because it allows minimally invasive surgery. The control and protection of the accessory nerve, sympathetic chain, and vertebral artery are the key to success. The exposure is safe if the anatomy is familiarized and if a rigorous step-by-step surgical technique is followed.

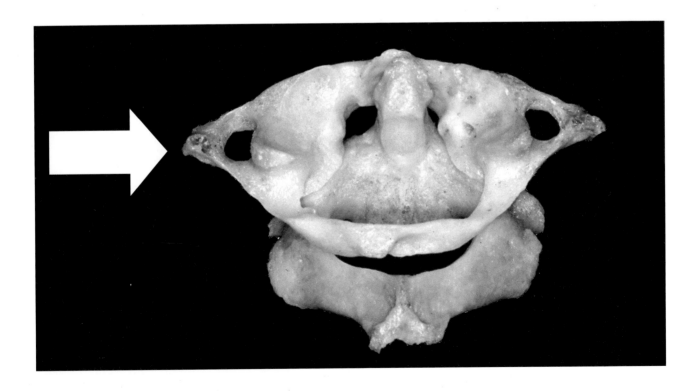

II. Procedure

Step-by-Step Cadaver Dissection

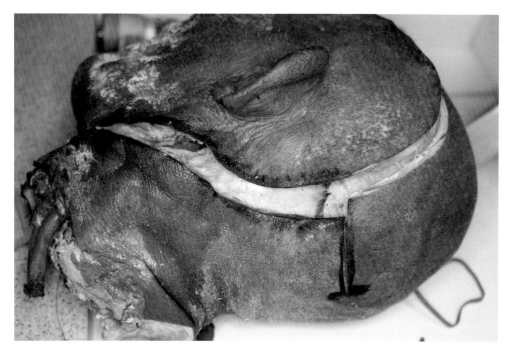

Figure 10-1. Incision

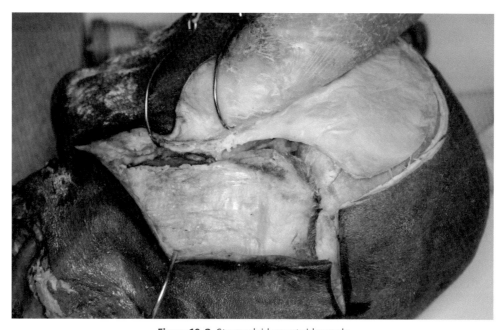

Figure 10-2. Sternocleidomastoid muscle

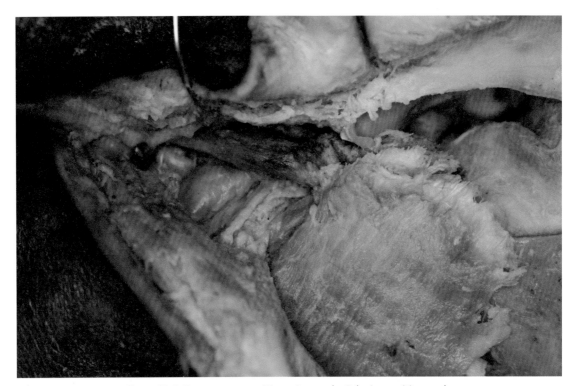

Figure 10-3. Accessory nerve, Digastric muscle, Splenius capitis muscle

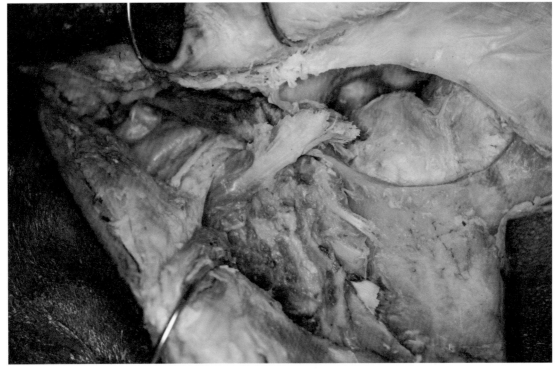

Figure 10-4. Longissimus capitis muscle

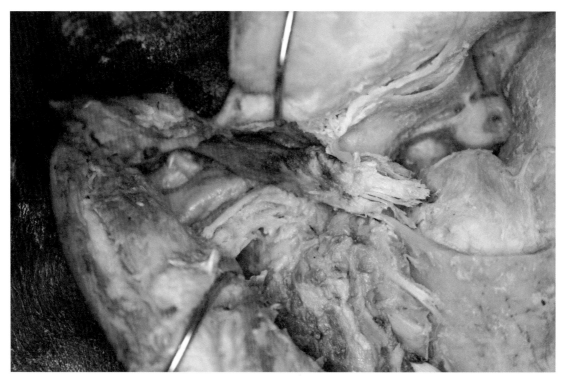

Figure 10-5. After longissimus capitis muscle retraction

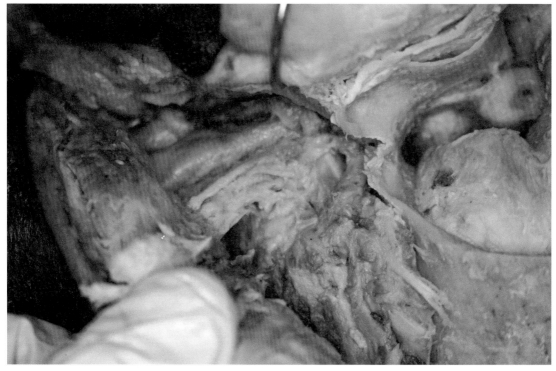

Figure 10-6. After digastric muscle retraction

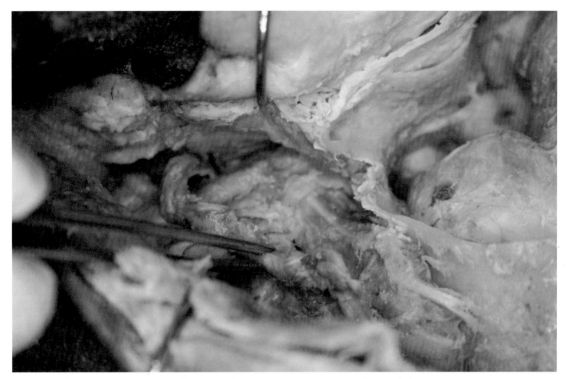

Figure 10-7. Occipital artery entering into external carotid artery

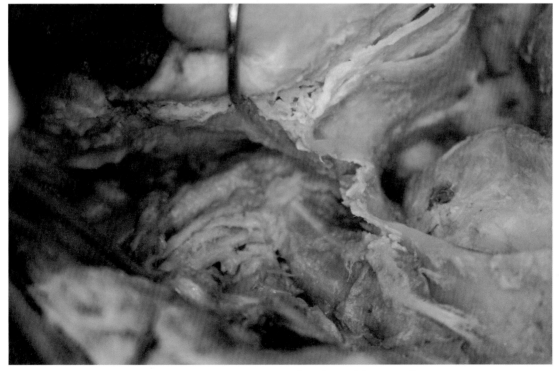

Figure 10-8. Superior oblique muscle, inferior oblique muscle

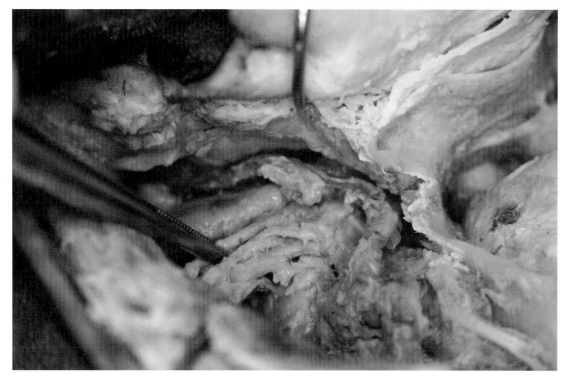

Figure 10-9. Accessory nerve underneath sternocleidomastoid muscle and on levator scapulae muscle

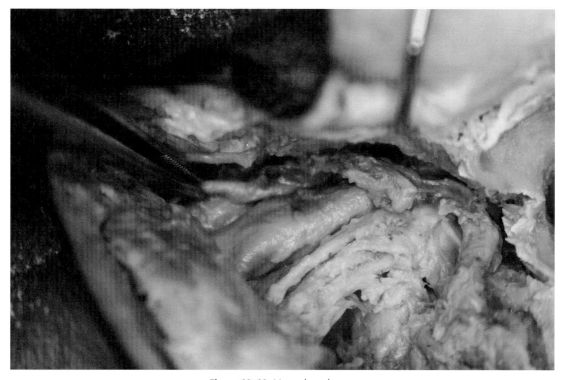

Figure 10-10. Hypoglossal nerve

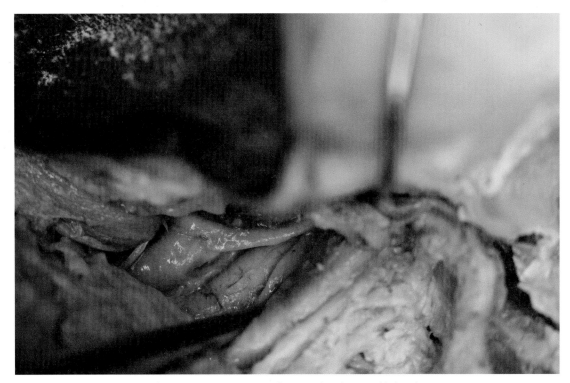

Figure 10-11. Vagus nerve after opening the carotid sheath

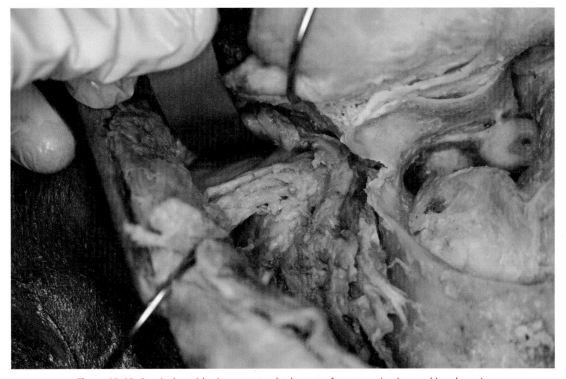

Figure 10-12. Surgical corridor into prevertebral space after retracting internal jugular vein

Indications

APPROACH	Anterolateral	Far lateral	Extended endoscopic endonasal
LOCATION	• extra-dural lesion • bone lesion • midline / lateral • C0-C7	• intra-dural lesion • lateral • lower clivus • C2	• extra- and intra-dural lesion • midline • above C2
EXAMPLE			

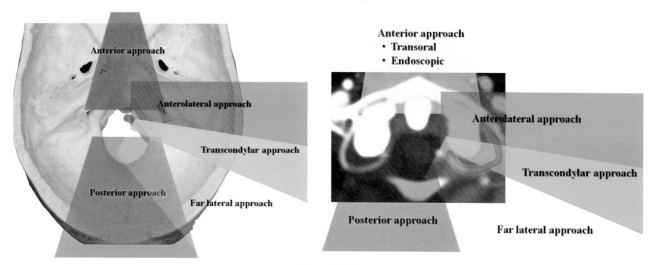

Figure 10-12.

Step-by-Step Surgery

1. Position

The patient is placed in supine position with 30-45° head rotation, in slight extension and fixed by a 3-pin Mayfield head holder. The head in slight extension facilitates in finding the margin of the sternocleidomastoid muscle. The more you rotate the head, the more the anterior arch of C1 disappears. The shoulder should not be elevated, if possible.

2. Incision

An L-shaped skin incision is made from the superior margin of the transverse sinus to the anterior margin of the sternocleoidomastoid muscle. The inferior margin of the skin incision can be extended according to the extent of the lesion as far down to C7.

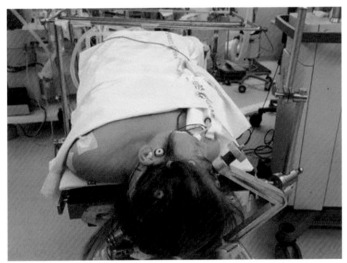

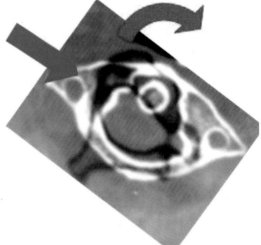

Figure 10-13.

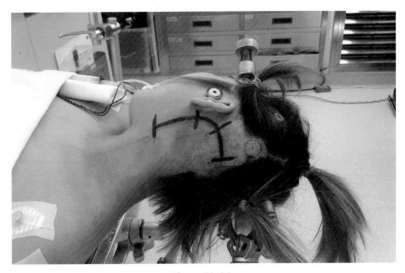

Figure 10-14.

3. Superficial Muscle Dissection

After the incision, the sternocleidomastoid muscle is identified and cut from its insertion point at the mastoid process and retracted in the medial direction.

4. Identification and Retraction of Accessory Nerve

The accessory nerve runs beneath the sternoclei-domastoid muscle from the transverse process of C1 in the direction of the levator scapulae muscle.

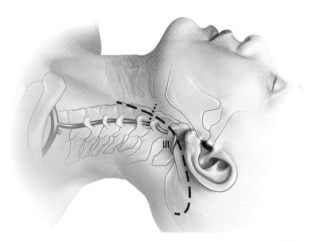
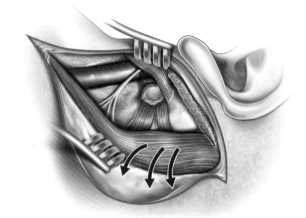

Figure 10-15.

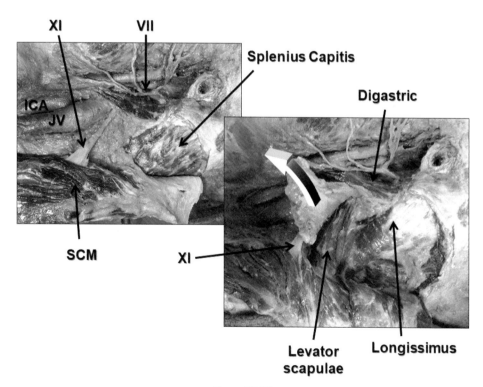

Figure 10-16.

Therefore, soft tissue dissection should be performed between the sternocleidomastoid muscle and the internal jugular vein and follow the posterior edge of the digastric muscle after palpating the transverse process of C1. Cranial nerve monitoring will also help locate the accessory nerve buried in the fat pad. Once the accessory nerve is identified, it is retracted with the fat pad in the inferior direction to expose the levator scapulae and splenius capitis muscles. The muscles are retracted in the medial direction to expose the longissimus capitis muscle, which is also retracted in the medial direction.

5. Deep Muscle Dissection and Vertebral Artery Mobilization

The digastric muscle is cut from its insertion point at the digastric ridge and retracted in the inferior direction to expose the rectus capitis lateralis muscle. The rectus capitis lateralis muscle is resected to expose the prevertebral space. The 3 muscles of the suboccipital triangle are cut from their insertion points and retracted to expose the venous plexus of the vertebral artery: the superior oblique muscle is cut from its insertion point at the superior nuchal line and retracted in the inferolateral direction, the rectus capitis major muscle is cut from its insertion point at the inferior nuchal line and retracted in the inferomedial direction, and the inferior oblique muscle is cut from its insertion point at the transverse process of C1 and also retracted in the inferomedial direction. The vertebral artery is mobilized with the venous plexus that encases it after opening the transverse foramen of C1.

The internal jugular vein is retracted in the medial direction with a self-retraining retractor to reach and resect any lesion in the prevertebral space through surgical window between the internal jugular vein and the transverse process of C1.

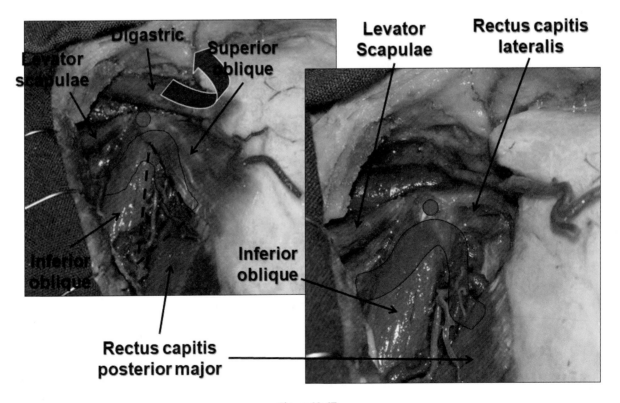

Figure 10-17.

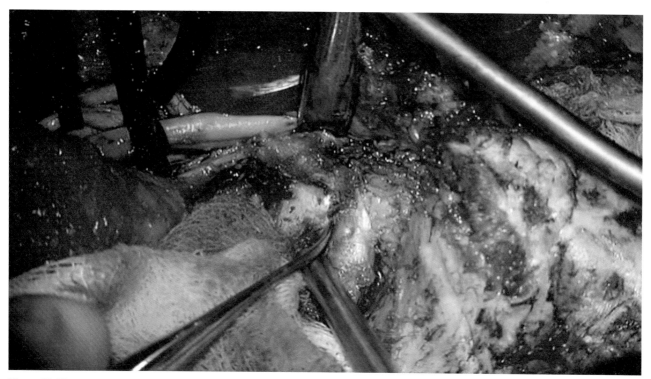

Figure 10-18.

Illustrative Case (video 10-1)

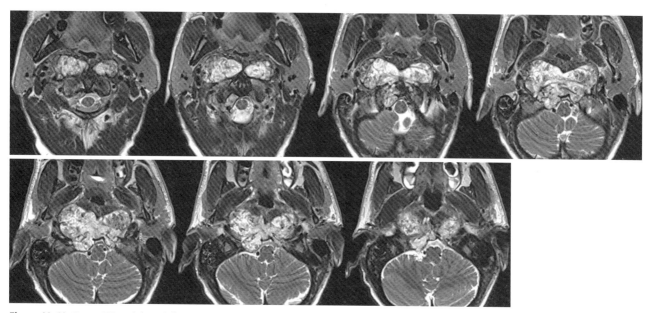

Figure 10-19. Preop T2-weight axial images of a clival chordoma

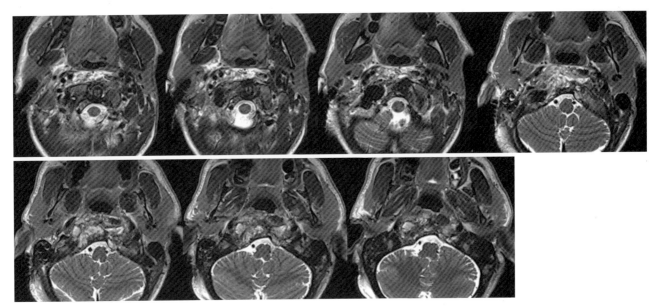

Figure 10-20. Postop T2-weight axial images of a clival chordoma

Video 10-1. An operation video of the Anterolateral approach.

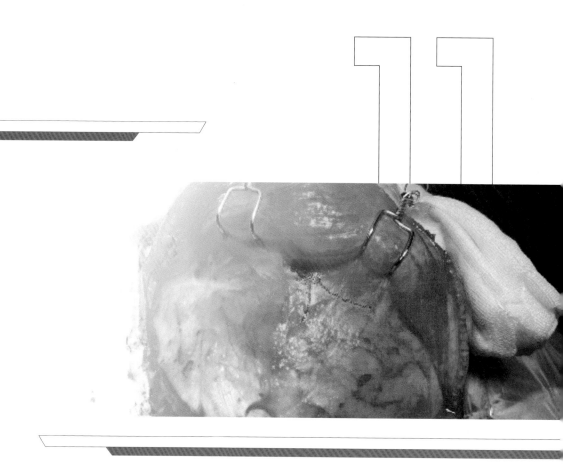

ONE-PIECE ORBITOCRANIAL APPROACH

Kyung-Sub Moon M.D., Ph.D., Shin Jung M.D., Ph.D.

I. Principle of the approach

The orbitocranial (OC) approach is a subtype of orbitozygomatic approach, which allows a steep angle of direct view to the base of the middle fossa and the roof of the orbit while minimizing brain retraction when compared to the usual perional or frontalateral approaches. With the removal of the orbital roof and anterior clinoid process, the entry angle is made shallower for exposure of the target. Unlike the orbitozygomatic approach that permits downward reflecting of temporalis muscle, the access of this approach can be limited to the lesion without extracranial extension into infratemporal fossa.

II. Indications

The indications of this approach are similar to those of the conventional orbitozygomatic approach. This approach gives excellent exposure of the lateral aspect of the sphenoid bone and access to the lesion of the intraorbital area, sphenoid ridge, planum, pituitary fossa, and upper part of the petroclival area. This approach is also useful for the parasellar or interpeducular lesions with lateral extension into the cavernous sinus or with considerable superior or posterior extension into temporoparietal or insular lobes. Combined with the extracranial or intracranial anterior clinoidectomy, it can provide longitudinal access to the entire internal carotid artery and its major branches and optic apparatus. This approach can be used for the skull base tumors that have invaded the frontal and middle cranial base, such as sphenoid/clinoid/cavernous meningioma, giant pituitary adenoma or craniopharyngioma, petrous apex or tentorial tumors. Due to the limitation in downward reflection of temporalis muscle, conventional orbitozygomatic approach seems to be superior for the lesion with extracranial extension into temporal base or infratemporal fossa.

III. Procedure

1. Position, skin incision, flap preparation

The patient is positioned supine and the head is turned 20 to 60 degrees (often 30-45) depending on the location of the lesion. Malar eminence (the body of the zygoma) is generally located on the highest point through the extension of the neck and inferiorly tilting of the vertex. A "question mark" (or simple curvy linear) skin incision is preferred. For sufficient exposure of the orbital rim and the frontal process of zygoma, the skin incision has to cross the midline about 2–5 cm and has to extend 0.5–1 cm caudal to the zygomatic arch. The inferior portion of the skin incision should be placed 1 cm anterior to the tragus due to prevent injury of the main trunks of the facial nerve. Supraorbital foramen, frontotemporale, frontozygomatic suture, and frontal process of zygoma are exposed and the nasion, zygoma, and zygomatic arch can be palpated. The superior orbital rim and frontotemporale are indicated in the photo (**Figure 11-1**).

2. Interfascial/subfacial dissection, detachment of temporalis muscle and periorbital

An interfascial or subfacial dissection (3-4 cm distance from orbital rim) is performed to remain underneath the branches of the facial nerve. The deep and the superficial layer of the temporalis fascia attaching to the orbital rim and the frontal process of zygoma are detached. The superficial layer is lifted toward the galea to expose the orbital rim and the frontal process of zygoma using fish hooks. The temporalis muscle is cut from the superior temporal line with 1 cm muscle cuff for preventing muscle retraction. The detachment of the periorbita is prepared from the base of the superior orbital rim just beyond the frontozygomatic suture line (**Figure 11-2**).

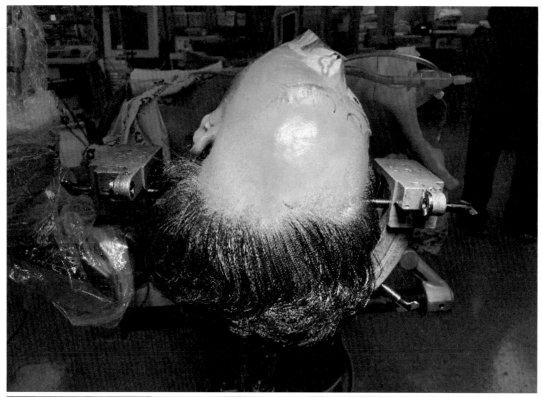

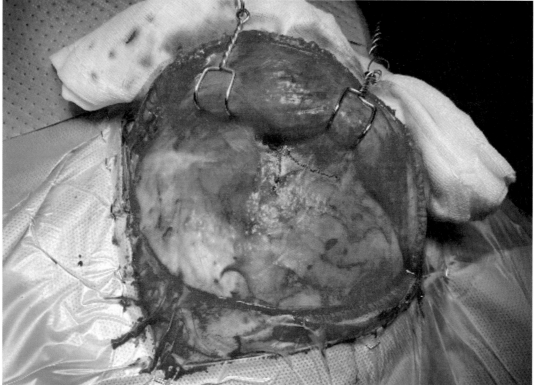

Figure 11-1.

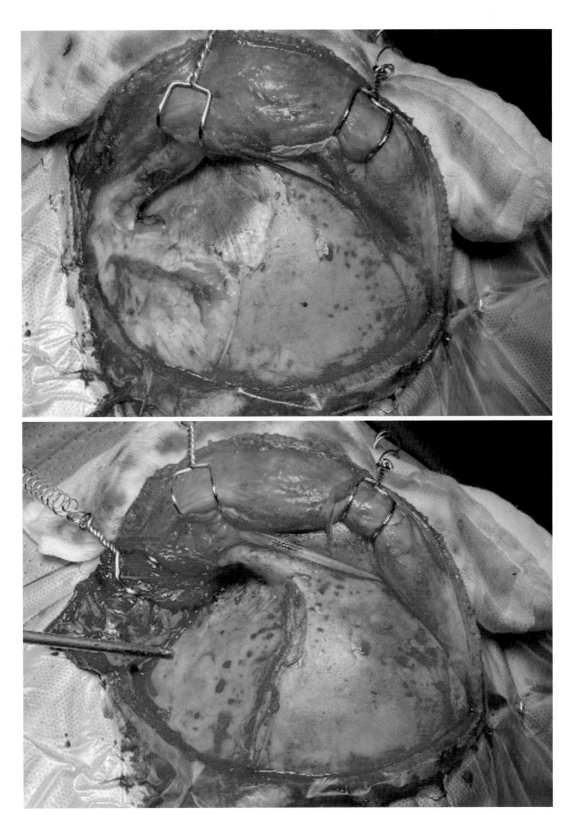

Figure 11-2.

3. Craniotomy

For one-piece OC craniotomy (**Figure 11-3**), the three burr holes are made including the McCarty's keyhole, which may be started over the anterior portion of frontosphenoid suture. It can be performed to cut with a 2-3 mm drill rather than a perforator to minimize damage to the dura mater and periorbita. McCarty's keyhole permits sufficient dissection of the dura superomedially and the periorbita inferolaterally. The first cut is made with an electric saw from the temporal hole through the parietal region to the orbital rim. Temporal base and sphenoid ridge bone can be thin enough by using a 2-3 mm drill & chisel. The frontal process of zygoma is cut with an oscillating saw just beyond the frontozygomatic suture. Superior orbital wall is cut with a chisel between the craniotomy margins (**Figure 11-4**).

Cotton pads are pushed into the dura and periorbita sides of the McCarthy hole to separate them from the skull and prevent injury. Fracture the lateral orbital wall between the two spaces with a chisel. Since the dura may be torn in the process of lifting the bone flap, the craniotomy is completed by carefully lifting the bone flap with dissection of the adhesion with the dura. Further drill-out of the temporal base and clinoid process can be adapted to this approach (**Figure 11-5**).

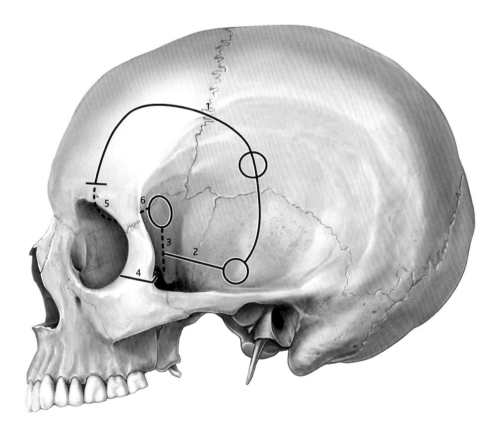

Figure 11-3. One-piece OC. After drilling 3 burr holes including the McCarty's keyhole, cutting off the 1st, 2nd, and 4th lines is performed with a saw or oscillating saw. And cutting off the 3rd and 5-6th lines follows using a drill or chisel through McCarty's keyhole to complete the craniotomy.

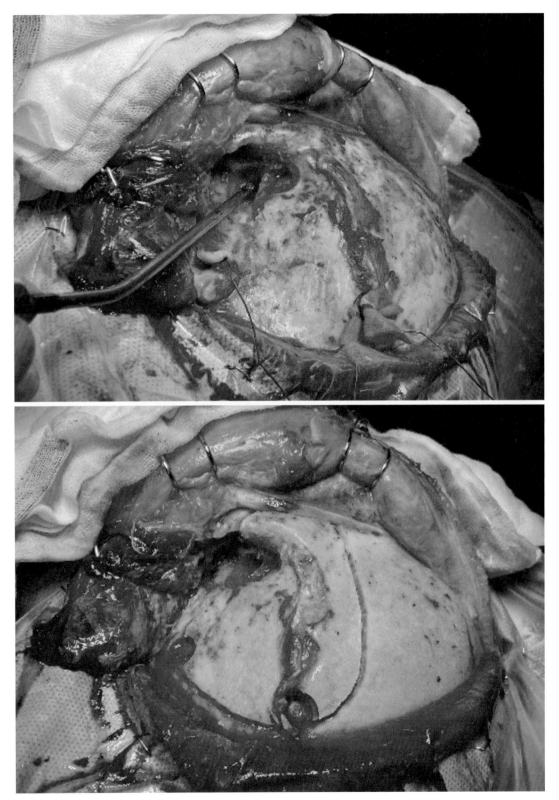

Figure 11-4.

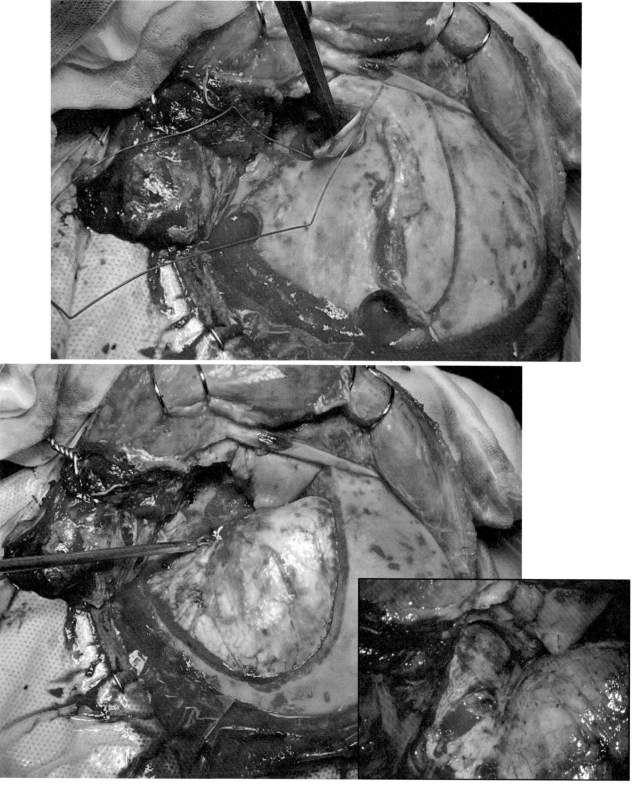

Figure 11-5.

[Case 1]

A 65-year-old female patient was admitted with visual impairment that had worsened for 1 year. Brain MRI revealed meningioma extending into the cavernous sinus in the left clinoid region (**Figure 11-6a**). The one-piece OC approach was decided to secure a wide corridor to the temporal base. After extradural partial removal of ACP, the Sylvian fissure was opened to minimize brain traction and the tumor was removed (**Figure 11-6b-d**).

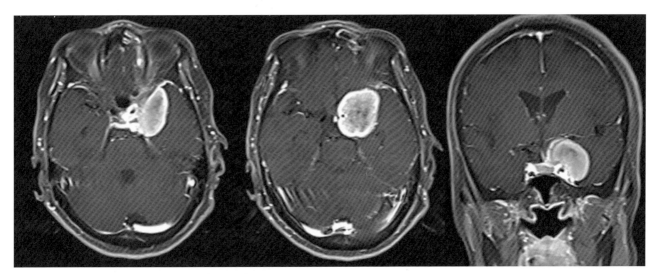

Figure 11-6a. Preoperative MRI showed left clinoid meningioma.

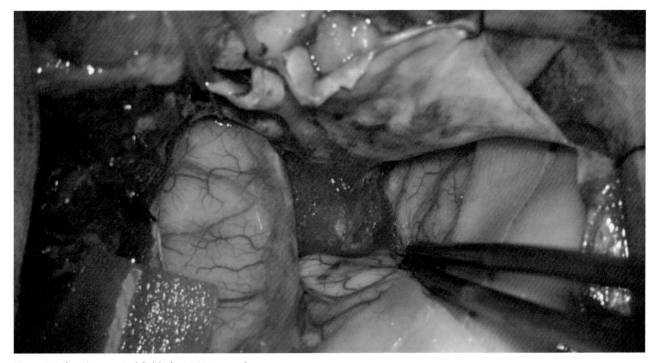

Figure 11-6b. Microsurgical field after ACP removal.

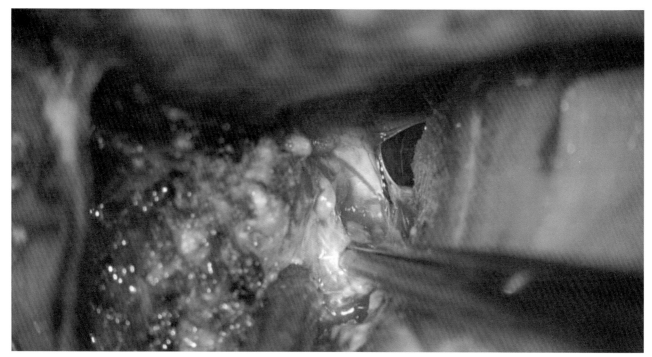

Figure 11-6c. Tumor removal with minimizing manipulation of optic nerve.

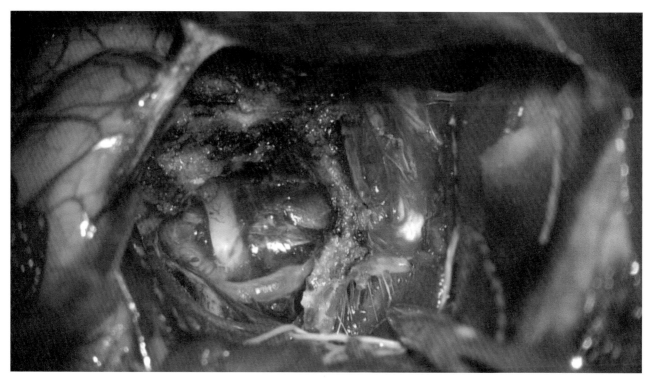

Figure 11-6d. Resection cavity after tumor removal. Oculomotor and optic nerve, P-com artery visualized. Some tumors tightly adhered to ICA main trunk and M1 and in the cavernous portion portion were left.

[Case 2]

A 62-year-old male patient was admitted with incidentally detected brain mass. Brain MRI showed a meningioma in the right clinoid region. (**Figure 7**) After usual one-piece orbitocranial approach with extradural partial removal of ACP, the Sylvian fissure was widely opened to minimize retraction and the tumor was removed (**Figure 11-7b, 2c**).

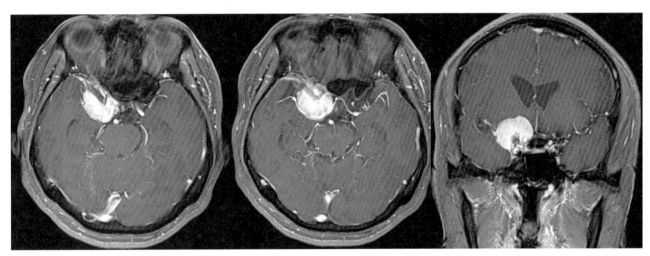

Figure 11-7a. Preoperative brain MRI. Rt. ICA was encased by right clinoid meningioma.

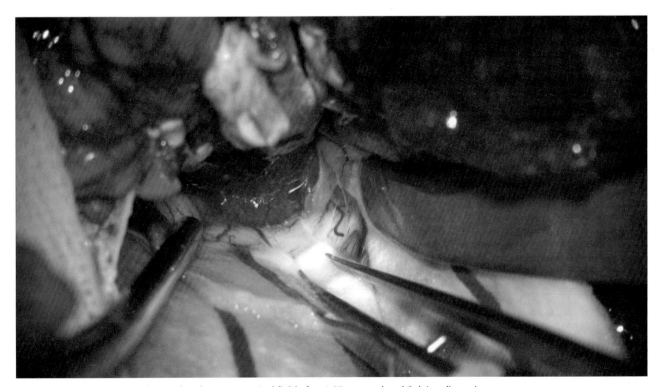

Figure 11-7b. A red mass is observed in the microsurgical field after ACP removal and Sylvian dissection.

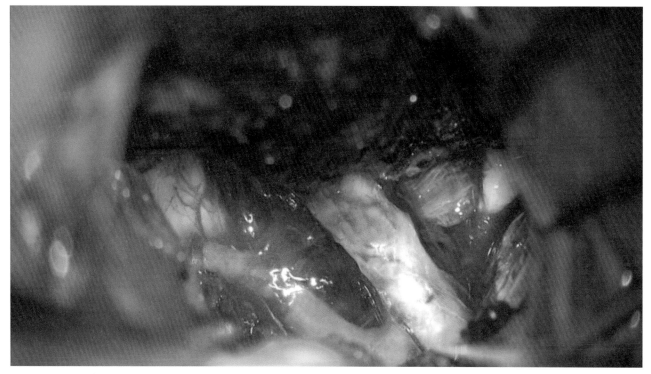

Figure 11-7c. Right ICA and ACA, optic nerve, and oculomotor nerve were found after tumor resection.

IV. Tips and Summary

1. Position with proper head tilting and vertex down so that the malar eminence is the highest point.
2. The skin should be incised enough to expose the frontal process of zygoma and the superolateral orbital rim. Perform interfascial or subfascial dissection of the temporalis muscle to prevent injury of the frontal branch of the facial nerve.
3. Detach the temporalis fascia from the orbital rim and the frontal process of zygoma with minimal use of monopolar cautery.
4. For one-piece craniotomy, burr-hole making on McCarty's keyhole is important.
5. Be careful in handling the chisel to cut the orbital roof after periorbital detachment and protection using cotton pads.
6. When the bone flap still is not entirely mobile after the final cut, cutting at the edge of the superior orbital rim and the frontal process of zygoma is confirmed and then gentle elevation of the bone flap can lead to the cutting of the final bony bridge with "crack sound".

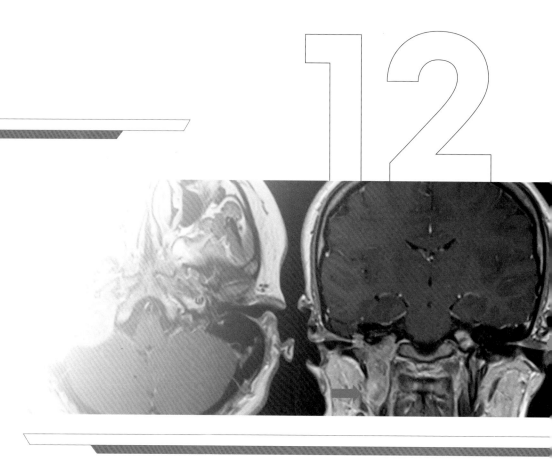

12

INFRATEMPORAL FOSSA APPROACH

In Seok Moon M.D., Ph.D.

I. Introduction

Infratemporal fossa approaches, in particular, require access to tumors through intertwined surrounding bones of the face and cranium (temporal bone, mandible, and zygoma, etc.), placing important cranial nerves and vessels at considerable risk of iatrogenic injuries.

Infratemporal fossa approach may provide access to lesions of the lateral skull base, including the jugular foramen, parapharyngeal space, pterygomaxillary fossa, clivus, nasopharynx, petrous apex, cavernous sinus, orbital apex, parasellar region, and the Infralabyrinthine compartment of the temporal bone.

These surgical approaches have evolved gradually over the past several decades and can be categorized historically as anterior (transfacial, transmaxillary, transoral, and transpalatal), lateral (transzygomatic and lateral infratemporal), or inferior (transmandibular and transcervical). Excellent descriptions have been provided by Fisch, who based his works on the need for facial nerve and internal carotid artery identification and preservation. The infratemporal fossa approach defined by Fisch is cosmetically superior to the anterior approach because there is no incision in the front of the face. However, it causes conductive hearing loss and causes temporary or permanent mild facial palsy.

Infratemporal fossa approaches are classified as type A, B, C, and D. Type A approach for access to the infralabyrinthine and petrous apex, Type B approach for lesions of the clivus, and Type C infratemporal approach for exposure of the nasopharynx. Type D is a modification of the type B and C approaches and is best suited for resection of lesions of the mid- and upper clivus, petrous apex, and cavernous sinus without violation of the middle ear or mastoid.

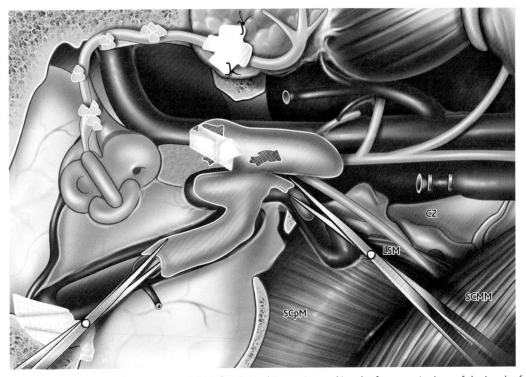

Figure 12-1. The type A approach provides exposure of the infralabyrinthine region and jugular foramen. Lesions of the jugular foramen, including glomus tumors, meningiomas, and schwannomas, can be removed through this approach. In the lateral approach, the facial nerve becomes the biggest obstacle to access to the tumor and the carotid artery or lower cranial nerves inwardly become the limitation for complete removal of the tumor. To complete removal and preservation of lower cranial nerve function, full exposure of tumor is essential. The proper rerouting of facial nerve and complete drilling of tympanic ring, fallopian canal, and perijugular bulb bone is very important.

II. Infratemporal fossa approach type A

1. Concept

The type A approach provides exposure of the in-fralabyrinthine region and jugular foramen. Lesions of the jugular foramen, including glomus tumors, meningiomas, and schwannomas, can be removed through this approach.

Case Example

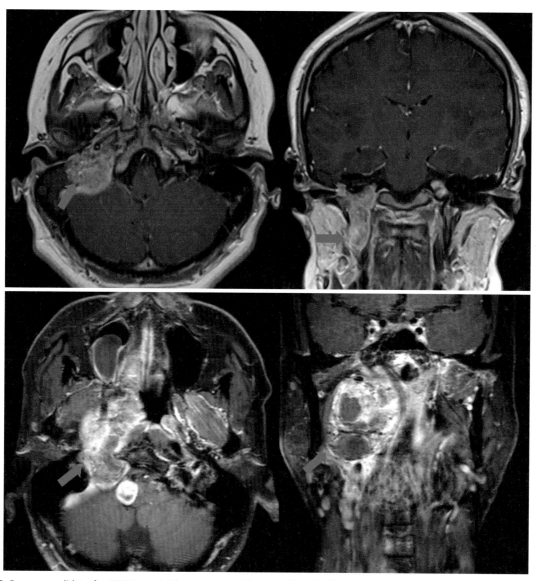

Figure 12-2. Proper candidate for ITFA type A. The upper panel is case of jugular foramen paragenglioma and lower panel is the case of jugular foramen Schwannoma. In the lateral approach, the facial nerve becomes the biggest obstacle to access to the tumor and the carotid artery or lower cranial nerves inwardly become the limitation for complete removal of the tumor. In paraganglioma, tumor is too hard and bloody to remove piecemeal manner. So facial nerve rerouting is the key procedure. Sigmoid sinus and jugular vein ligation are needed. But in Schwannoma, we can remove the tumor in piecemeal manner, fallopian bridge technique can be an alternative for avoiding facial palsy.

2. Positioning and skin incision

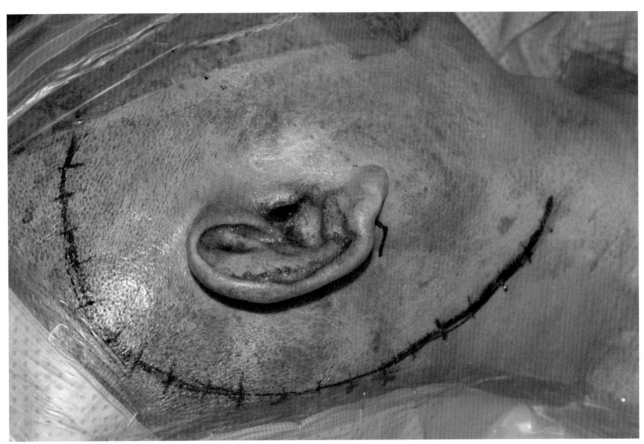

Figure 12-3. Patient's head position with the zygoma as the highest point on the operative field. The vertex of the patient's head is tilted slightly toward the floor. This maneuver maximizes the effect of gravity retraction on the temporal lobe. Curvilinear scalp incision. It starts immediately posterior to the ear and finally descends near to the level of the zygomatic arch, about 1 to 2 centimeters in front of the tragus. The curvilinear incision mobilizes the muscle effectively away from the operative working zone.

3. Flap elevation & external auditory canal (EAC) management

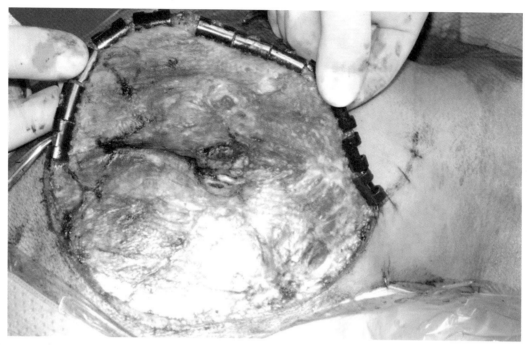

Figure 12-4a. External auditory canal shoud be cut at eht level of cartilage-bone junction. Wide undermining of the anterior edge of the skin creates an anteriorly based musculoperiosteal flap that aids closure.

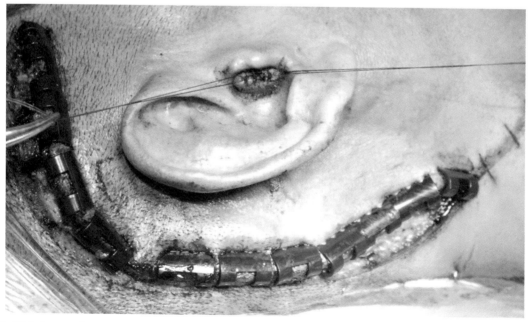

Figure 12-4b. EAC closure. The cuff of canal skin is dissected from the cartilage surrounding the meatus and everted. This everted skin is closed with interrupted 4-0 vicryl sutures. Inner side was reinforced using cartilage or muscle pedicle.

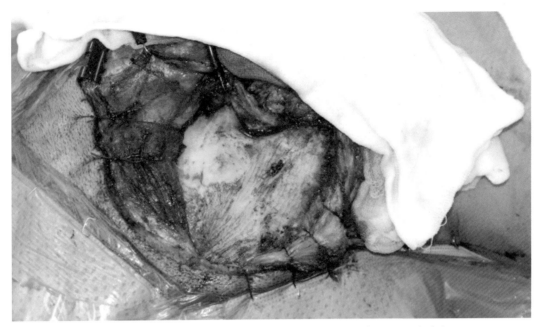

Figure 12-4c. A periosteal flap is elevated from the undersurface and retraction can serve better surgical view.

4. Bone work

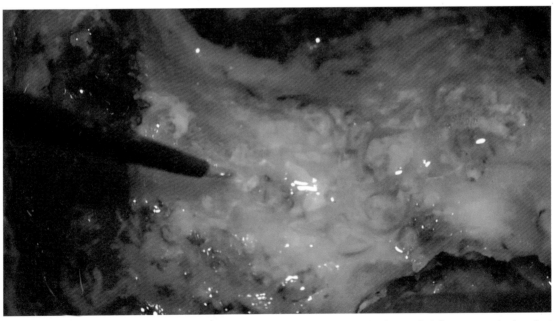

Figure 12-5a. Identification of Facial Nerve. The main trunk in temporal bone is identified using facial nerve monitoring device and is skeletonized. The superficial lobe of the parotid gland need to be dissected and main trunk should be exposed. Neck Dissection can be done in this step or later. If done in this step, the sternocleidomastoid muscle (SCM); the posterior belly of the digastric muscle the internal jugular vein; the ICA and ECA, and CNs IX, X, XI, and XII are identified. Loops or umbilical tapes are placed around the great vessels. See Figure 12-7b.

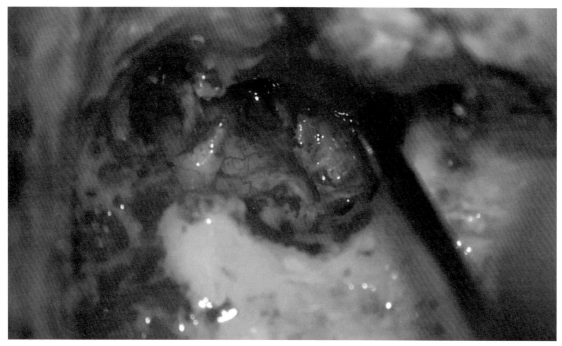

Figure 12-5b. Removal of middle ear structure. The remaining posterior bony external auditory canal and skin are removed. After separation of Incudo-malleolar joint separation and resection of tensor tendon, the tympanic membrane need to be completely removed. A radical mastoidectomy, including removal of the mastoid tip is performed. In this process, sigmoid sinus is skeletonized and uncapped.

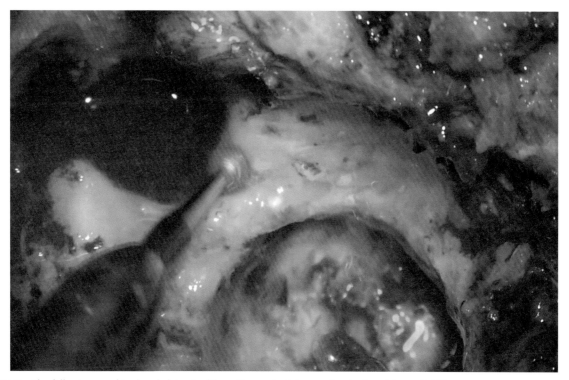

Figure 12-5c. The fallopian canal is also skeletonized from the geniculate ganglion to the stylomastoid foramen.

5. Facial Nerve Rerouting

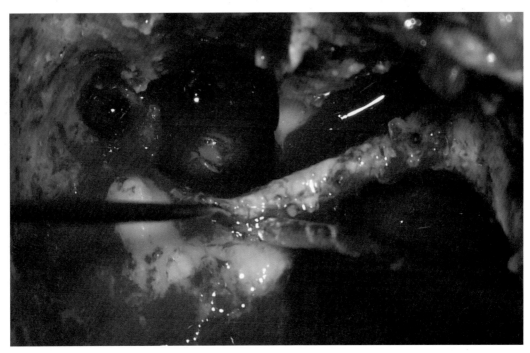

Figure 12-6a. Anterior transposition of facial nerve. After a new fallopian canal is drilled in the zygomatic root superior to the Eustachian tube, facial nerve is freed from originanl fallopian canal. It's fibrous attachments are composed of venous plexus and much bleeding can be happen. Massive bleeding control and rough manipulation can damage the nerve. Meticulous elevation from its original position is needed.

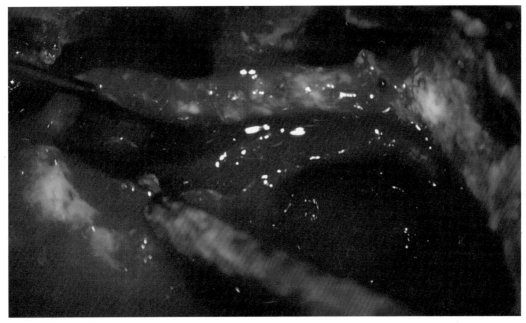

Figure 12-6b. Next, a vertical incision is made in the parotid gland to create a tunnel to house the repositioned nerve. Facial nerve is anterior reposed and Fibrin glue may be applied to the nerve to secure it to its new position.

6. Tumor Exposure

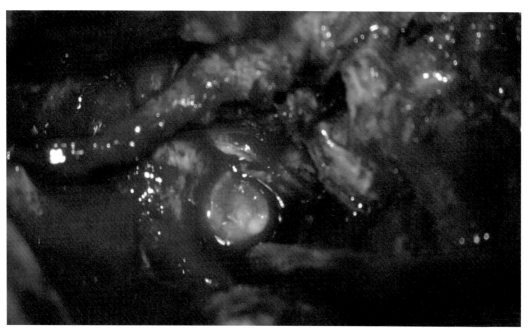

Figure 12-7a. After securing the facial nerve in new position, original fallopian canal and bony structure under the canal is drilled to expose the tumor. Bony structure medial to the digastric muscle, superior to atlas, posterior and lateral to jugular bulb should be maximally drilled.

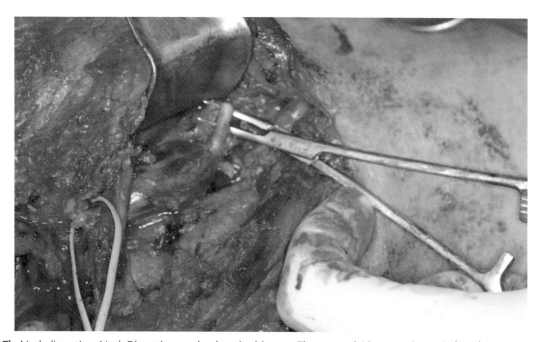

Figure 12-7b. Neck dissection. Neck Dissection can be done in this step. The sternocleidomastoid muscle (SCM); the posterior belly of the digastric muscle; the internal jugular vein; the ICA and ECA, and CNs IX, X, XI, and XII are identified. Loops or umbilical tapes are placed around the great vessels.

7. Tumor removal

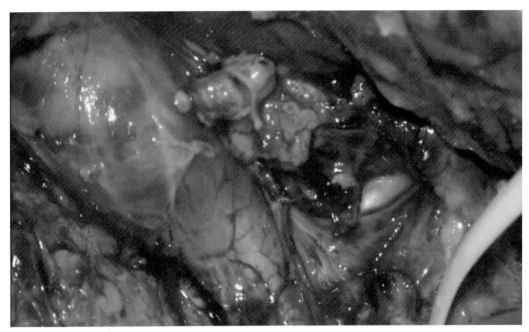

Figure 12-8a. The internal jugular vein and external carotid artery are ligated in the neck and divided. The jugular vein is then dissected and elevated superiorly as far as the intradural extension of the tumor toward the jugular bulb. It may be necessary to pull the vein under CN XI to prevent injury.

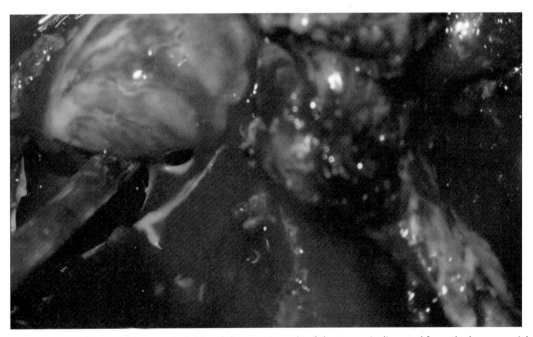

Figure 12-8b. Jugular vein and sigmoid sinus are incised and the superior pole of the tumor is dissected from the lower cranial nerves and otic capsule. The lateral wall of the jugular bulb is also opened and resected along with tumor. Bleeding from communicated sinuses can be done using packing with coagulation materials. The anterior pole of the tumor is mobilized from the petrous ICA. During this step, bleeding from the caroticotympanic branches is controlled with bipolar cauterization. If the adventitia has been invaded, a small portion of tumor is left adherent to the ICA for separate resection.

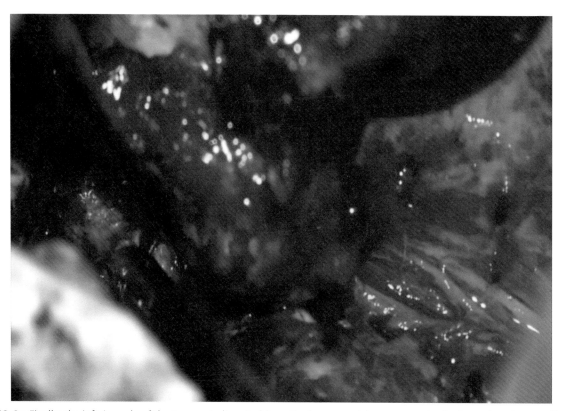

Figure 12-8c. Finally, the inferior pole of the tumors is dissected from the lower cranial nerves, starting in the neck and proceeding superiorly to the jugular bulb. The extradural tumor can now be separated sharply from the intradural portion. Large intradural extensions of tumor cannot be resected in one stage using the type A infratemporal fossa approach.

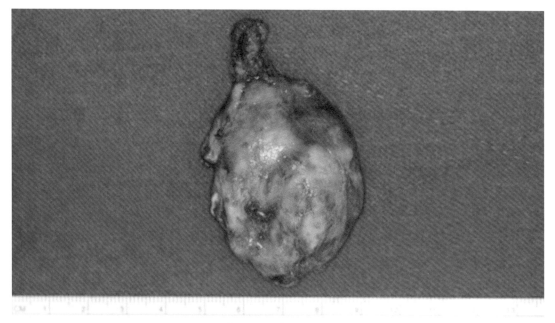

Figure 12-8d. Specimen.

Closure

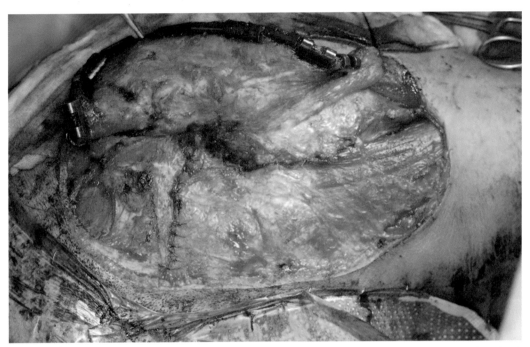

Figure 12-9a. The Eustachian tube is plugged with harvested temporalis muscle tissue. The dura is reapproximated as closely as possible. Dural defects can be closed with a temporalis fascia graft. The wound cavity is packed with abdominal fat.

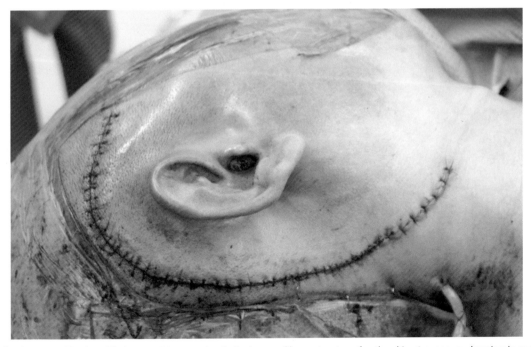

Figure 12-9b. The wound is closed in layers with a running locked monofilament suture for the skin. A pressure dressing is applied at the end of the procedure.

III. Infratemporal fossa approach type B & C

1. Concept

The type B approach is designed for parapharyngeal tumor, petrous apical tumor, and midclival tumors. The type C approach is an anterior extension of type B and provides access to the pterygopalatine fossa, parasellar region, and nasopharynx.

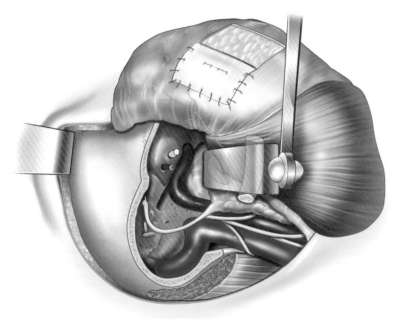

Figure 10. The type B approach is designed for petrous apical and midclival tumor. The type C approach is an anterior extension of type B and provides access to the pterygopalatine fossa, parasellar region, and nasopharynx.

Case Example

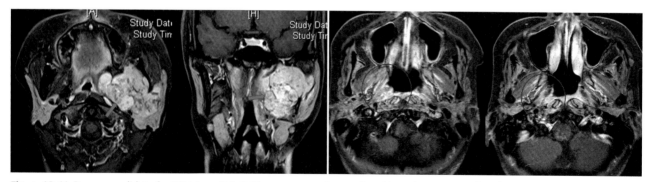

Figure 12-11. Proper candidate for ITFA type B & C. The upper panels are adenoid cystic carcinoma (ACC) originated from parotid gland and the candidate for ITFA B. The lower panels are nasopharyngeal cancer and the candidate for ITFA C.
In the case of ACC from parotid gland, of course we need to perform total parotidectomy, but the tumor involves pterygoid fossa, only parotidectomy is not enough. Tumors of the parapharyngeal space can be resected using ITFA B which have classically been thought as unresectable. The Fisch type C approach has been used both as a primary treatment and in the salvage surgery for nasopharyngeal cancer, but now more used as salvage aim.

2. Positioning, skin incision, and Zygomatic arch cutting

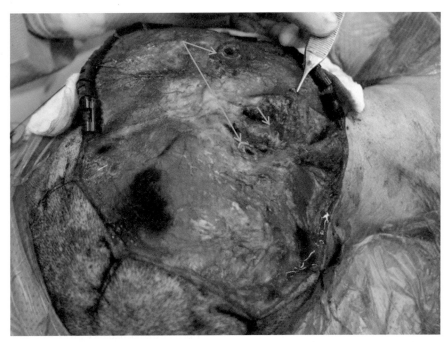

Figure 12-12a. A wide postauricular area and the entire ipsilateral neck are prepared and draped. The patient's head is turned away from the lesion. During the surgery facial and lower cranial nerves are monitored continuously. The large postauricular C-shaped incision is extended into the neck two fingerbreadths below the angle of the mandible and almost to the midline at the level of the thyroid cartilage. The ear is dissected anteriorly, and the ear canal is transected at the cartilage-bone junction. EAC closure. The cuff of canal skin is dissected from the cartilage surrounding the meatus and everted. This everted skin is closed with interrupted 4-0 vicryl sutures.

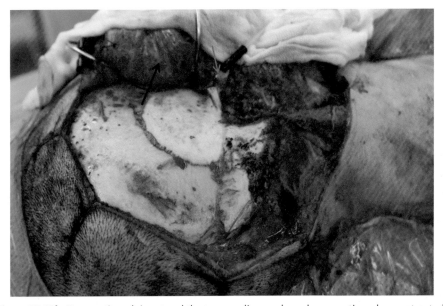

Figure 12-12b. Zygomatic arch is cut and the temporalis muscle and zygomatic arch are retracted.

3. Bone work

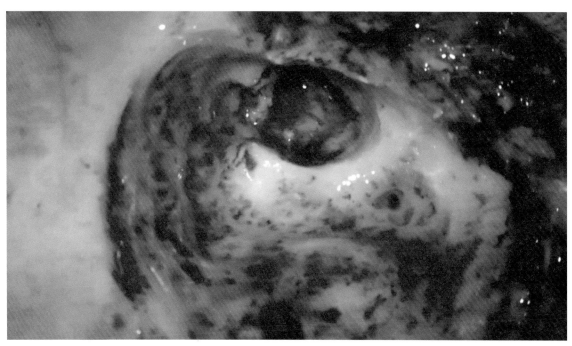

Figure 12-13a. Removal of middle ear structure. The remaining posterior bony external auditory canal and skin skin are resected. After separation of Incudo-malleolar joint separation and resection of tensor tendon, the tympanic membrane need to be completely removed. A radical mastoidectomy performed. In this process.

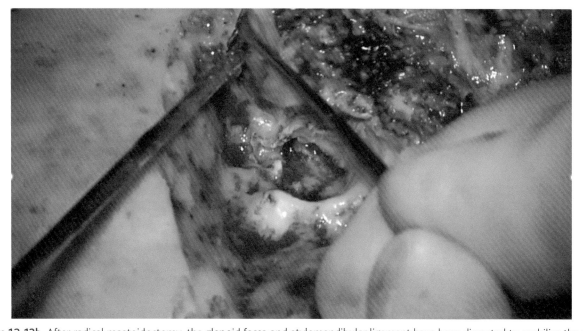

Figure 12-13b. After radical mastoidectomy, the glenoid fossa and stylomandibular ligament have been dissected to mobilize the mandibular condyle.

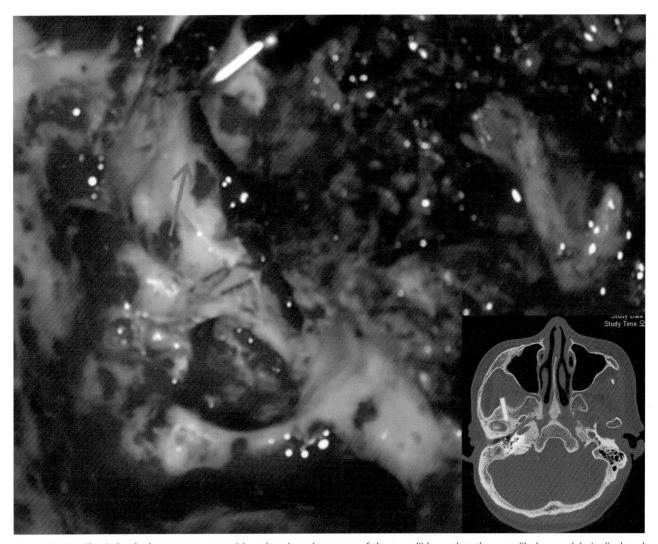

Figure 12-13c. Elastic hooked retractors are positioned against the ramus of the mandible so that the mandibular condyle is displaced anteriorly (arrow). This retraction makes resection of the mandibular condyles unnecessary. After all its attachments have been cut, the styloid process is fractured and resected with a rongeur. This maneuver exposes the fibrous tissue covering the carotid canal. Resection of this tissue, followed by the drilling of the residual anterior wall of the external auditory canal, completes exposure of the vertical portion of the ICA.

4. Identification and ligation of landmarks

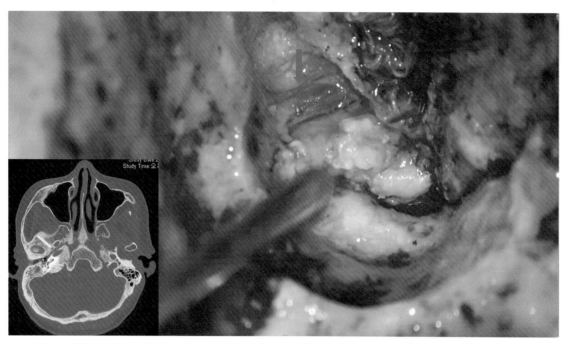

Figure 12-14a. Middle Meningeal artery (arrow) is exposed and cut to access to the bony Eustachian tube.

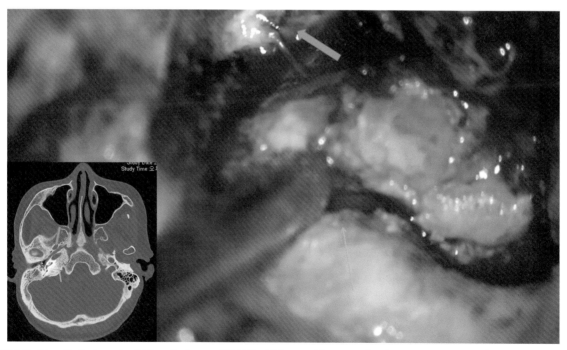

Figure 12-14b. Mandibular branch of trigeminal nerve (CN V3, thick arrow) is exposed and cut to access to the bony Eustachian tube. It is followed by residual tympanic temporal bone drilling with a diamond bur until tumor or catilaginous Eustachian tube are identified. The Internal carotid artery (thin arrow) is posterior limitation.

5. Tumor exposure & removal

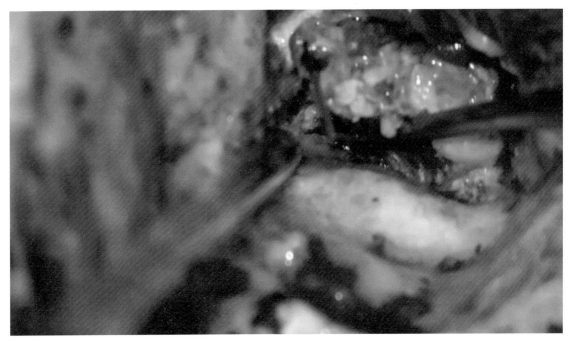

Figure 12-15a. Tumor in nasopharynx is be removed enbloc with surrounding tissue extending to the contralateral nasopharyngeal wall. Superior landmark is tegmen and tumor can be dissected from skullbase bone.

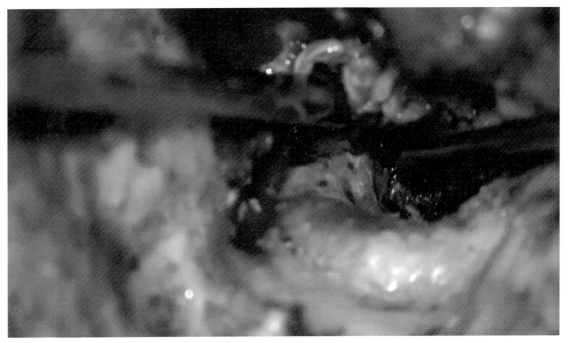

Figure 12-15b. Tumor in nasopharynx is be removed enbloc with surrounding tissue extending to the contralateral nasopharyngeal wall. Antero-medial landmark is mucosa or resenmullar fossa and tumor can be dissected following catilaginous Eustachian tube and can meet the mucosa of Rosenmuller fossa

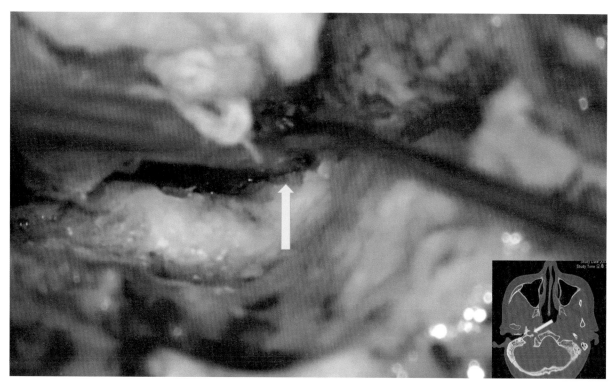

Figure 12-15c. Tumor in nasopharynx is be removed enbloc with surrounding tissue extending to the contralateral nasopharyngeal wall. Postero-inferior landmark is horizontal segment of internal carotid attery and tumor can be dissected following this landmark.

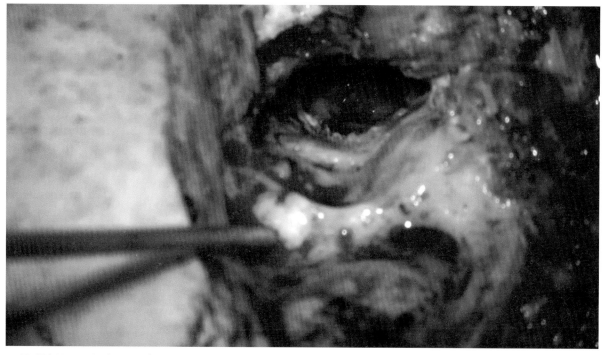

Figure 12-15d. Tumors in the nasopharynx is removed enbloc with surrounding tissue extending to the contralateral nasopharyngeal wall.

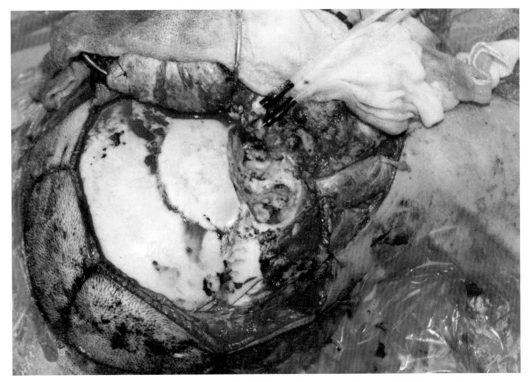

Figure 12-16a. Eustachian tube is exposed and dissected to access the tumor in the nasopharynx.

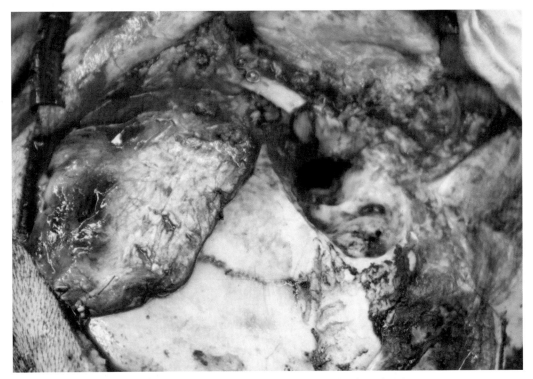

Figure 12-16b. Zygomatic bone should be repositioned to keep facial contour.

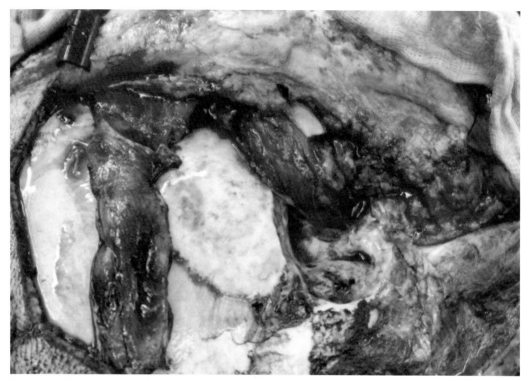

Figure 12-16c. We reinforce the defect with rotational muscle flap of temporalis muscle. Fibrin glue is applied.

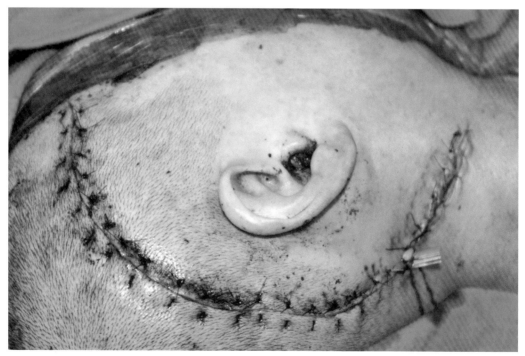

Figure 12-16d. The wound is closed in layers with a running locked monofilament suture for the skin. A pressure dressing is applied at the end of the procedure

REFERENCES

1. Fisch U, Fagan P, Valavanis A. The infratemporal fossa approach for the lateral skull base. Otolaryngol Clin North Am 1994;17(3):513-52.

2. Franklin DJ, Moore GF, Fisch U. Jugular foramen peripheral nerve sheath tumors. Laryngoscope 1989;99(10):1081-87.

3. Zhang M, Garvis W, Linder T, Fisch U. Update on the infratemporal fossa approaches to nasopharyngeal angiofibroma. Laryngoscope 1997;108:1717-23.

4. Choi JY, Lee WS. Curative surgery for recurrent nasopharyngeal carcinoma via the infratemporal fossa approach. Arch Otolaryngol Head Neck Surg 2005;131(3):213-6.

5. Banuchi V, Kraus DH. The infratemporal fossa approach to the lateral skull base and parapharynx. Oper Tech Otolayngol Head Neck Surg 2014;25(3):254-8.

6. Ramina R, Maniglia JJ, Fernandes YB, Paschoal JR, Pfeilsticker LN, Neto MC, et al. Jugular foramen tumors: diagnosis and treatment. Neurosurg Focus 2004;17(2):E5.

7. Chung HJ, Moon IS, Cho H-J, Kim C-H, Sharhan SSA, Chang JH, et al. Analysis of surgical approaches to skull base tumors involving the pterygopalatine and infratemporal Fossa J Craniofac Surg 2019;30(2):589-95.

8. Moon IS, Kim J, Lee H-K, Lee W-S. Surgical treatment and outcomes of temporal bone chondroblastoma. Eur Arch Otorhinolaryngol 2008;265(12):1447-54.

9. Chung SM, Kim HS, Jung J, Lee H-K, Lee WS. Clinical presentation and management of jugular foramen paraganglioma. Clin Exp Otorhinolaryngol 2009;2(1):28-32.

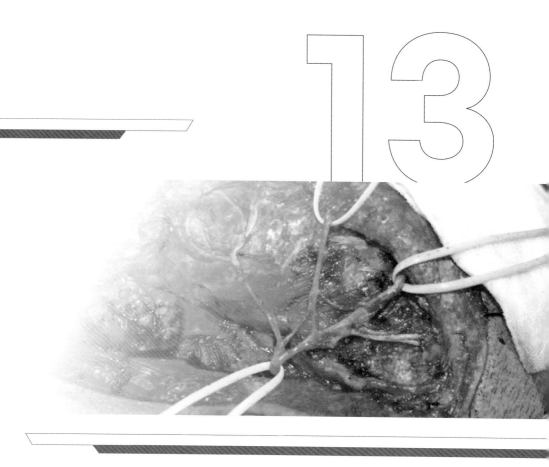

THE PARAPHARYNGEAL SPACE (HIGH CERVICAL SPACE) APPROACH

Han Su Kim M.D., Ph.D.

I. Introduction

A generic term, 'the high cervical space' is referred to as 'the parapharyngeal space'. The parapharyngeal space (PPS) is a potential deep area in the upper lateral neck. The PPS is described as an inverted pyramid with the floor of the pyramid at the skull base and the apex at the level of the greater cornu of the hyoid bone.[1] It is limited posteriorly by the prevertebral aponeurosis and musculature of C1–C2 and C3, medially by the pharyngobasilar fascia and the superior pharyngeal constrictor muscle and laterally by the medial pterygoid muscle, the ascending branch of the jaw, the superficial cervical fascia and the submandibular gland.(Figure 13-1) The PPS is usually divided into two compartments by the styloid process and its related muscle bundles. The pre-styloid compartment is mainly occupied by a deep lobe of the parotid gland and fat, while the post-styloid compartment contains vital organs; the internal carotid artery, internal jugular vein, cranial nerves IX to XII, cervical sympathetic chain, fat and lymph nodes. In recent literature, this well-known classification has been given a different designation. The previously named pre-styloid space is now called the real PPS, while the post-styloid space is now designated the carotid space.[2]

Different tumors can arise from all of the different structures present in the PPS. The tumors of the PPS constitute less than 1% of all head and neck tumors, and almost are benign tumor (80%); almost half of them originate from the salivary glands (40–50%), while the rest arise from nervous structures (20%) or are enlarged lymph nodes (15%). Approximately, 20% are malignant tumors. Of all PPS tumors, pleomorphic adenoma is the most common.[3] Tumors of the parapharyngeal space (PPS) are rare and almost benign, they have many challenging issues both in diagnosis and treatment. Preoperative pathologic assessment of the PPS tumors is insufficient, due to the complex anatomical barrier of this space making it inaccessible.

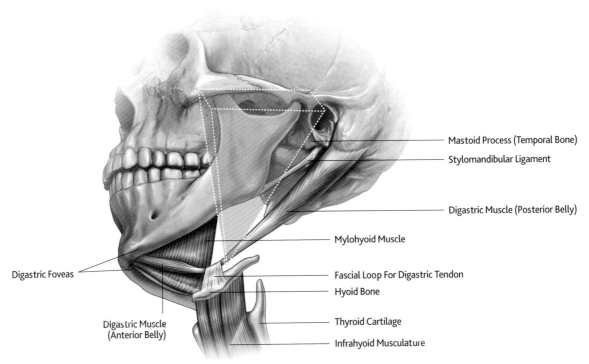

Figure 13-1. The parapharyngeal space and its relative anatomies. The PPS is an inverted cone-shaped space that extends from the skull base to the hyoid bone.

Labels in figure:
Mastoid Process (Temporal Bone)
Stylomandibular Ligament
Digastric Muscle (Posterior Belly)
Mylohyoid Muscle
Fascial Loop For Digastric Tendon
Hyoid Bone
Thyroid Cartilage
Infrahyoid Musculature
Digastric Foveas
Digastric Muscle (Anterior Belly)

II. Selection of approach

Many different approaches to the PPS have been described and this reflects the intrinsic difficulty in surgical access to this space. The parotid gland and the submandibular gland are the outermost barriers to PPS. The parotid gland also contains the facial nerve which is the bothersome barrier too. The most constant barrier is the mandible. Therefore, various approaches had been developed to bypass the barriers.

The transcervical approach was first described while the transcervical-transparotid approach is the most widely used. For small lesions, transoral approaches could be used. A transparotid approach is the preferred surgical method of removal of deep parotid lobe tumors; A transparotid approach is essentially necessary for dissecting and transposing branches of the facial nerve to gain adequate access. Therefore, a transparotid approach may keep facial nerves safely under direct identification but cause iatrogenic injuries during dissection of the nerves.

In most cases of the prestyloid parapharyngeal space tumors, a transcervical approach is safe and offers excellent direct visualization of the tumor and all critical neurovascular structures.[4] The important anatomies, the carotid artery, the internal jugular vein, and lower cranial nerves (CN10, CN11, CN12) are easily identified during cervical dissection at the level of I and II. Transcervical approach is the most accepted approach for the parapharyngeal space space masses arising from the minor salivary glands and in cases when the transparotid approach alone is insufficient for the removal of large deep lobe parotid tumors. The parapharyngeal space can be accessed by mobilization of the submandibular gland.[4]

For large tumors involving the deep parotid lobe and extending into the prestyloid parapharyngeal space, a combined transparotid-transcervical approach is usually warranted, both to gain adequate access and to perform the surgery safely with limited morbidity.[4] The transparotid approach offers good surgical field for safe identification of the facial nerve and all its branches, while the transcervical approach gives excellent direct approaches to manipulate all critical neurovascular structures within the parapharyngeal space.

Historically, deep lobe parotid tumors and even parapharyngeal space masses have been tried to remove transorally. A transoral approach is controversial and abandoned by many surgeons with prejudice of the inadequate exposure, neurovascular risk, the wound healing problems, and the tumor spillage. A transoral approach was usually combined with the transparotid or the transcervical approach (dual approaches).[5] Technological advances in robotics and increasing use of robotic-assisted surgery in the oropharynx and the parapharyngeal space are sparking a renewed interest in the transoral route as a potential minimally invasive approach for tumor removal in carefully selected cases.[4,6]

All of above approaches have anatomical limitations caused anteriorly by the mandibular ramus and posteriorly by the temporal bone and styloid apophysis. If needed, the transcervical approach may be combined with a trans-mandibular modification. Different mandibulotomies, have been developed to enhance exposure of this space for safer tumor removal. The mandibulotomy approach presents a wide surgical field, but it has also many other limitations and morbidities. Therefore, the mandibulotomy approach is used when the tumor is malignant and invades to the skull base.

III. Procedures

1. Patient preparation

The patient was placed in the supine position (**Figure 13-2**). Naso-tracheal intubation may occasionally be preferred in selected cases. An intubation through the nostril contralateral to the tumor permits complete closure of mouth with approximation of the teeth potentially allowing better access to deep lobe tumors that have parapharyngeal extension. In the case of the transparotid approach, NIMS (nerve integrity monitoring system) might be placed for nerve monitoring. You must notice the use of NIMS to an anesthesiologist before anesthesia. Therefore, an anesthesiologist

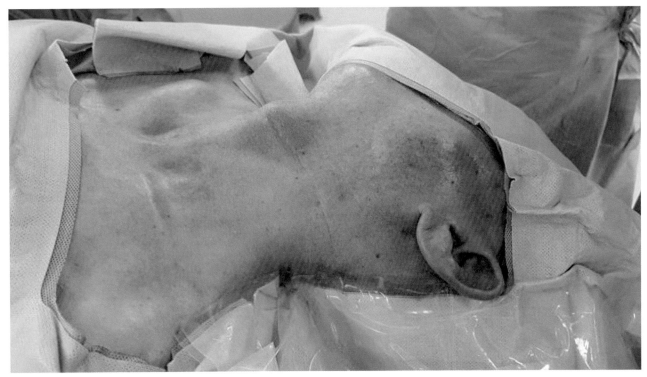

Figure 13-2. Patient's position and surgical drape. A shoulder roll was placed to extend the neck. A whole neck, the auricle and the half of the face are draped.

should not use a muscle relaxant or less.

2. Skin incision

Skin incisions vary depending on the approaches. A skin incision for transcervical approach is made, extending from the mastoid tip to the greater cornu of the hyoid bone 2-3 finger-widths below the body of the mandible, so that the inferior aspect of the submandibular gland may be easily identified. You must keep in mind that the lowest branch of facial nerve runs along the lower border of the mandible, therefore neck incision should be made at enough distance from the border (**Figure 13-3a**). Modified Blair incision is widely used for the transparotid approach. Briefly, an incision in front of the ear curves behind the angle of the mandible and extends anteriorly two fingerbreadths beneath (3 cm) the lower border of the jaw. In case of transparotid-transcervical approach, an extended incision, mentioned above, is made over

the submandibular gland. For trans-mandibular approach, lip splitting incision should be made. This incision is usually extended from cervical incision (**Figure 13-3b**).

3. Skin flap elevation

Subplatysmal skin flaps are elevated by sharp dissection. In the case of transcervical approach, the flaps are raised up to the level of the mandible and down to the superior aspect of the thyroid cartilage. It is careful not to cause thermal and electric injury to the marginal mandibular branch of the facial nerve. Direct visual identification of the marginal mandibular branch of the facial nerve and raise up with skin flap together are safer and improve mobilization of the submandibular gland.

For the transparotid portion, skin flaps are raised in the supra superficial muscular aponeurotic system (SMAS), in a similar plane to facelift procedure.

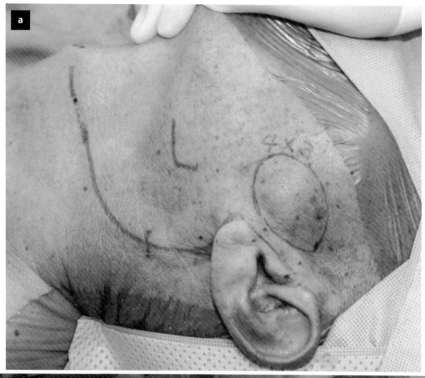

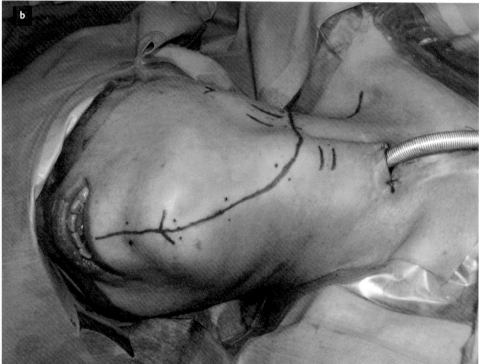

Figure 13-3. Skin incisions for the transcervical-transparotid approach (a) and the transmandibular approach (b). For the transcervical approach conventional neck incision, a curvilinear skin incision beginning at the mastoid tip, is used and it can be extended with the modified Blair incision for the transparotid approach (a). The transcervical incision is combined with a lip slitting incision for the transmandibular approach (b).

The SMAS is a superficial fascial layer that extends throughout the cervical facial region, and all facial nerve branches always run just deep to the SMAS. In the lower face, the SMAS invests the facial muscles and is continuous with the platysma muscle. The key maneuver is to transition from a supra-SMAS dissection to a strictly subplatysmal dissection in the neck as the SMAS transitions into the platysma muscle below the mandible. This is a critical maneuver to help protect the marginal mandibular and cervical branches of the facial nerve as they course deep to the platysma muscle.[4] A "cobble-stoning" of fat on the undersurface of the flap is a good indicator of proper elevation plane. It is helpful to diminish risk of symptomatic Frey's syndrome by making a thicker skin flap. After skin flap elevation, place 2-0 silk "stay sutures" into the

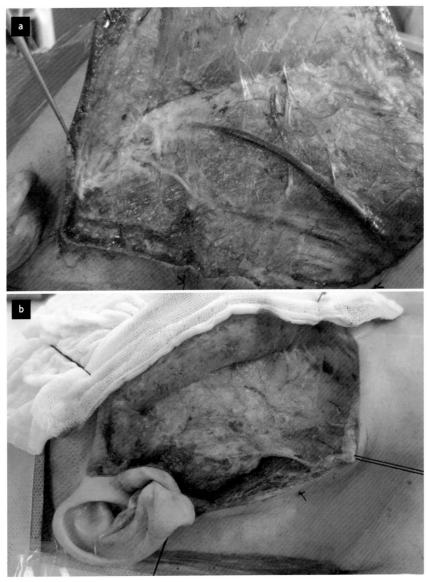

Figure 13-4. Skin flap elevation. Subplatysmal skin flaps are elevated by sharp dissection. In the case of transcervical approach, the flaps are raised up to the level of the mandible and down to the superior aspect of the thyroid cartilage (a). For the transparotid portion, skin flaps are raised in the supra superficial muscular aponeurotic system (b).

ear lobe for posterior retraction and stay sutures into the cheek flap for anterior retraction (**Figure 13-4**).

4. Transcervical approach

After skin flap elevation, the submandibular gland is sharply dissected and mobilized anteriorly as much as possible. The small vessels and connective tissues around the gland are ligated and dissected, which will help mobilize the gland. Some surgeons prefer to remove the submandibular gland altogether; however, removal of the gland does not markedly improve access to the parapharyngeal space and is not necessary in most cases.[7]

The hypoglossal and lingual nerves are always identified for protection during dissection to the parapharyngeal space. The hypoglossal nerve can be iden-

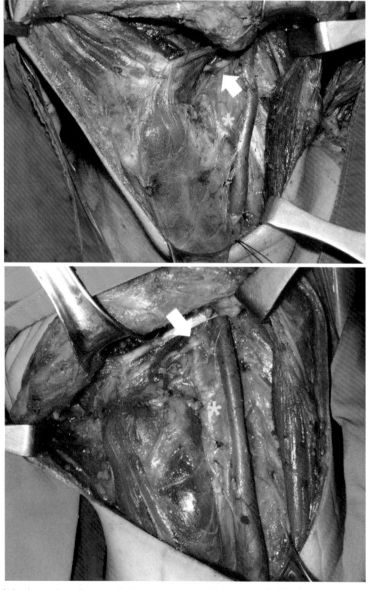

Figure 13-5. Identification of the hypoglossal nerve during the transcervical approach. The hypoglossal nerve (white arrow) runs cross over the carotid artery (yellow asterisk) and into the mylohyoid muscle.

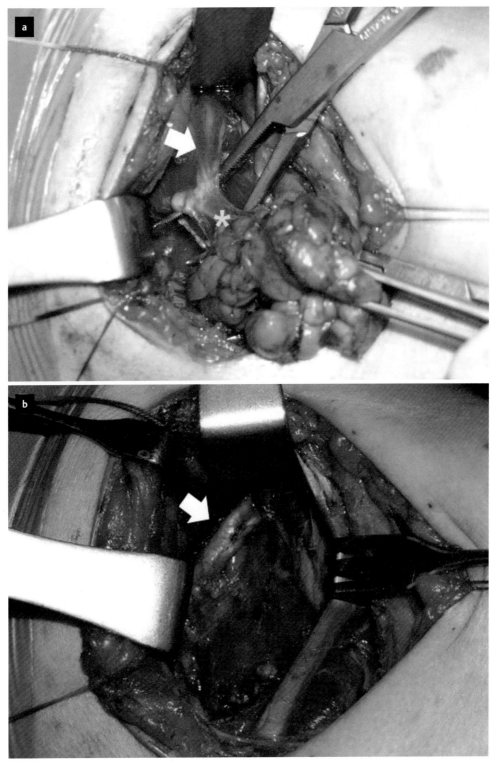

Figure 13-6. Identification to the lingual nerve. The lingual nerve (white arrow) is connected with the submandibular gland via the submandibular ganglion (yellow asterisk, a). After removal of the submandibular gland, the lingual nerve is located superiorly when the mylohyoid muscle and the digastric muscle are retracted (b).

tified in its inferior position as it crosses the carotid artery laterally and the posterior belly of digastric muscle medially (**Figure 13-5**). The hypoglossal nerve is also identified after retraction of the submandibular gland, where the nerve dives under the mylohyoid muscle medially. The lingual nerve is found situated between the submandibular gland and the hyoglossus muscle. It is easily exposed when the mylohoid muscle is retracted anteriorly and the submandibular gland is retracted inferiorly (**Figure 13-6**).

The mandible is then retracted upward, and PPS is exposed (**Figure 13-7**). When the inferior portion of the tumor can be palpable, fibrous tissues over the tumor are then dissected carefully. After exposure of the tumor, it is bluntly dissected from the parapharyngeal space with a sponge or the surgeon's finger (**Figure 13-8**). This is performed carefully in the space between the mandible laterally and the constrictor muscles medially and the mobilized submandibular gland an-

teriorly. The dissection of the upper part of the tumor with a sponge or finger must be performed carefully and with gentle pressure, so as to not push through the constrictor muscles and violate the mucosal lining.

Extension of the transcervical approach to include complete removal of the submandibular gland and division of the digastric muscle can facilitate access to the parapharyngeal space (**Figure 13-9**).[4] If it is difficult to remove the tumor with blunt dissection, you should suspect a malignant infiltration or an inflammatory process. The dissection of the upper part of the tumor with a sponge or finger must be performed carefully and with gentle pressure, so as to not push through the constrictor muscles and violate the mucosal lining.

After removal of the tumor, complete bleeding control and thorough saline irrigation are mandatory. A drain is left in the parapharyngeal space and closure is performed in a layered fashion.

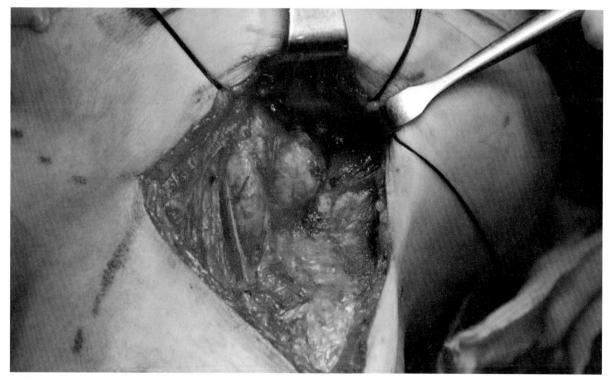

Figure 13-7. The exposure of parapharyngeal space via transcervical approach. When the mandible is retracted upward, the inferior portion of the parapharyngeal space can be exposed.

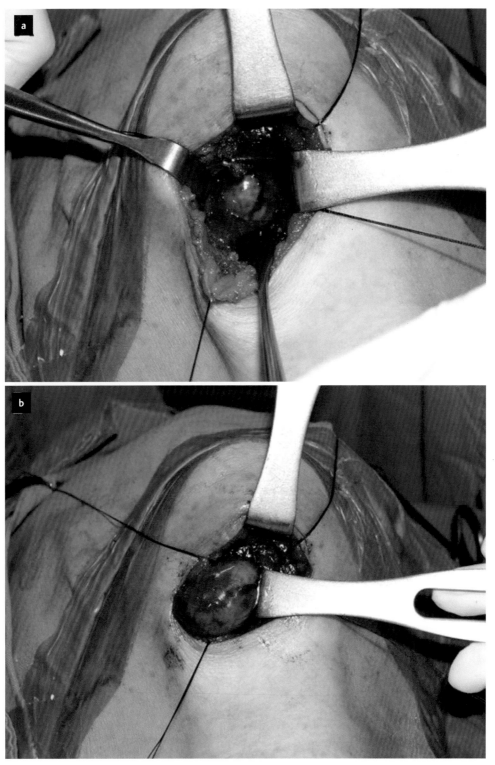

Figure 13-8. The exposure of the tumor and blunt dissection. When the inferior portion of the tumor is exposed, fibrous tissues over the tumor are then dissected carefully (a). The tumor is bluntly dissected from the parapharyngeal space with a sponge or the surgeon's finger (b).

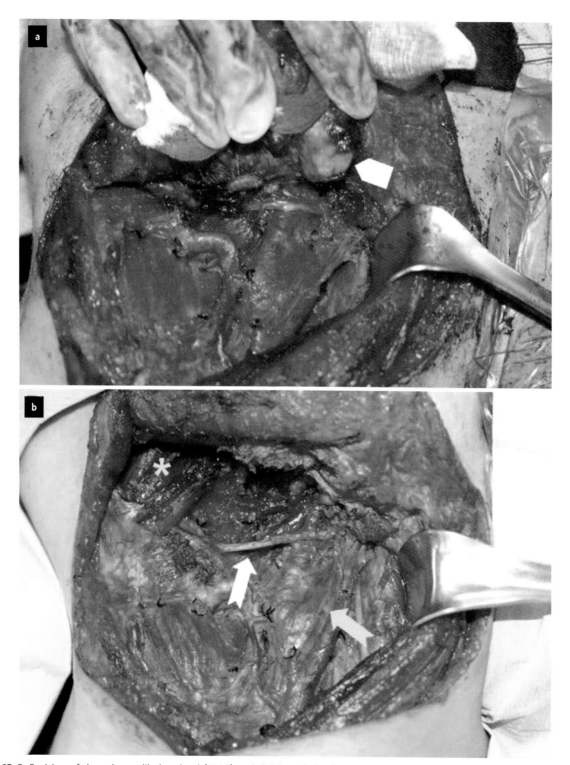

Figure 13-9. Excision of the submandibular gland (SMG) and division of the digastric muscle. In the case of large masses, a removal of SMG and the resection of the posterior belly of the digastric muscle is necessary to improve the exposure of parapharyngeal space. (a) Before removal of the SMG (arrow head), (b) After removal of the SMG and the resection of the digastric muscle. The mylohyoid muscle (asterix), the carotid artery (yellow arrow) and the hypoglossal nerve (white arrow) are well exposed.

5. Transparotid approach

Major concerns in the transparotid approach is to identify and protect the facial nerve and all its branches. The main trunk of the facial nerve is usually identified in a standard fashion using surgical landmarks; The tragal pointer, the insertions of the digastric muscle and sternocleidomastoid muscles (SCM) into the mastoid tip are exposed through 'mobilization' of the parotid gland (**Figure 13-10**). The greater auricular nerve may be divided for enough mobilization by dissecting between the tail of the parotid gland and SCM. If a posterior branch is identified, it often can be pre-served (**Figure 13-11**). After identification of the main trunk of the facial nerve, a superficial parotidectomy is performed by dissecting the superficial lobe away from all the facial nerve branches (**Figure 13-12**). After completion of a superficial parotidectomy, the deep portion of the parotid gland can be removed. Nerve hooks or loupes are used to elevate the facial nerve. A small, sharp scissors is used to cut the fascial connections from the gland to the nerve, completely freeing and isolating the entire course of the facial nerve from the main trunk at the level of the styloid foramen to the periphery over the masseter muscle (**Figure 13-13**).

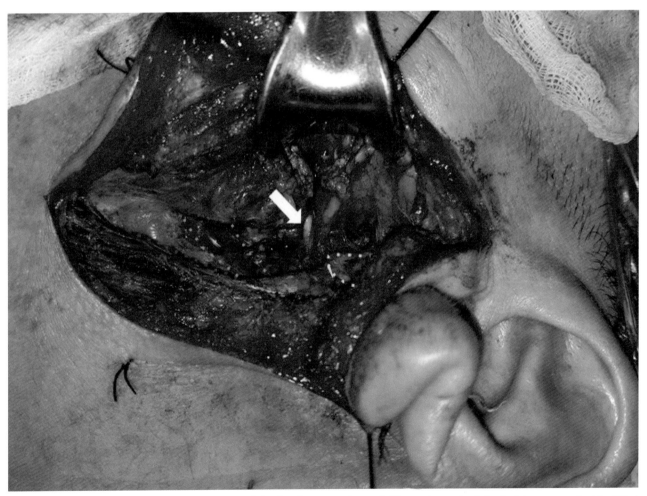

Figure 13-10. Surgical landmarks for identification of the facial nerve main trunk. The main trunk of the facial nerve can be identified between the tragal pointer (yellow line) and the posterior belly of the digastric muscle (green line). The parotid gland should be freely mobilized from the anterior border of the sternocleidomastoid muscle (red line) to expose the tragal pointer and the digastric muscle.

The tumor located in PPS is then dissected free between : now mobilized the facial nerve branches. This is performed with a gentle and meticulous technique to minimize trauma and traction injury to the delicate facial nerve branches (**Figure 13-14**).[4] In many cases only those facial nerve branches that interfere with exposure of the tumor can be mobilized and displaced to minimize morbidity (**Figure 13-15**). However, when a malignant tumor invades the facial nerve and the mobilization of the facial nerve is impossible, it is often forced to divide the facial nerve. In case of nerve division, cable graft must be performed. There are

many reconstructive methods for facial nerve reanimation. The author prefers the great auricular nerve (GAN) graft.[8] Because the GAN is easily harvested in the same operation field and the caliber of the GAN is similar to that of the facial nerve (**Figure 13-16**). The tumor is completely removed, and hemostasis is assured. A drain is left in the operation field, and the surgical wound is closed in layer by layer fashion.

The dissection and division of the stylomandibular ligament (with or without styloid process) also allows for greater anterior displacement of the mandible. After this procedure, most benign tumors within the

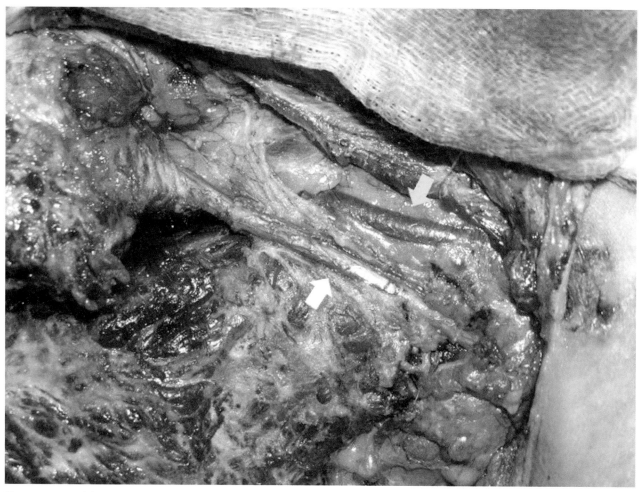

Figure 13-11. Mobilization of the parotid gland from the sternocleidomastoid muscle. The greater auricular nerve (white arrow) and the external jugular vein (yellow arrow) can be preserved during the mobilization of the parotid gland tail.

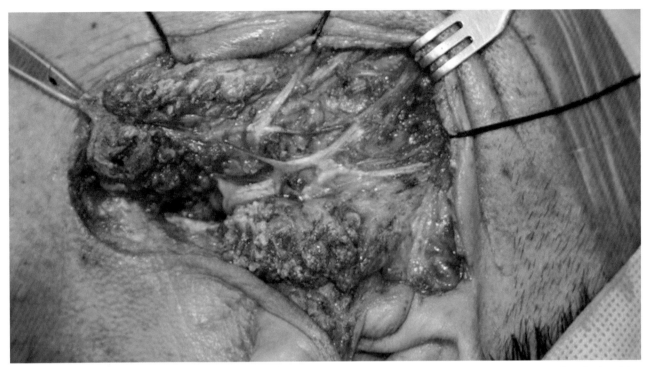

Figure 13-12. The transparotid approach. Superficial parotidectomy is performed and all the facial nerve branches are identified and dissected free from the deep lobe of the parotid gland.

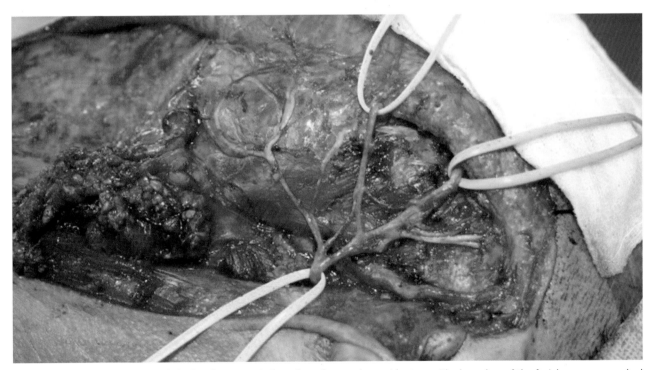

Figure 13-13. The identification of the facial nerve main branches after total parotidectomy. The branches of the facial nerve are marked with colored band for easily identification during surgical procedures.

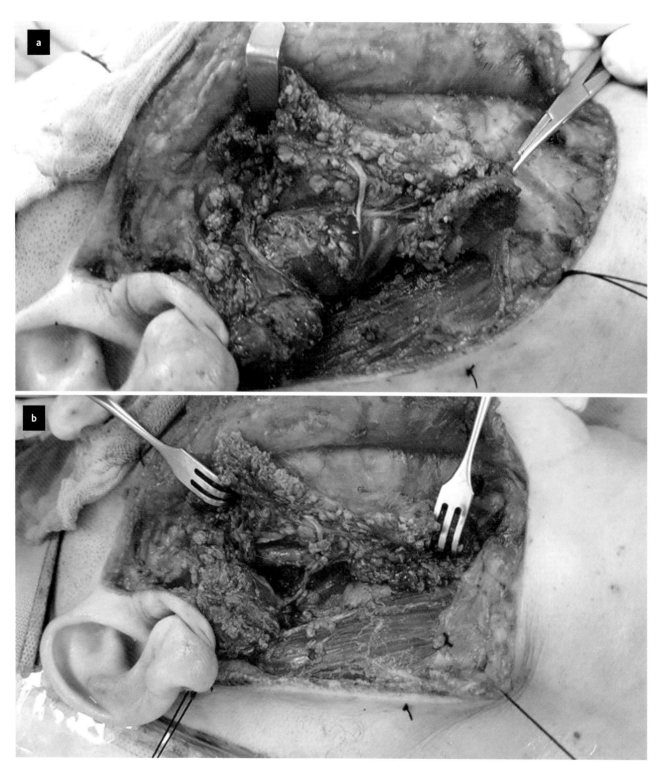

Figure 13-14. Transparotid approach. A parapharyngeal space tumor was exposed after a superficial parotidectomy (a). The tumor was removed with careful preservation of all branches of the facial nerve (b).

parapharyngeal space are easily dissected with finger dissection.

6. Transparotid-transcervical approach

Skin incision is done in a similar fashion combining transparotid and transcervical incision using neck skin crease. Once the skin flaps are raised, the transparotid approach is usually performed first as previously described. A complete superficial parotidectomy is usually not performed, but the lower half of the super-

ficial lobe of the parotid gland is removed for identification of lower branches of the facial nerve. This is necessary to combine with a transcervical approach without any traumatic injury to the nerve branches, especially the marginal mandibular nerve.

The transcervical approach is then undertaken, and all critical neurovascular structures should be identified; the external carotid artery and its branches could be ligated with stick-ties and divided for exposure of the tumor. The dissection is then carried around the

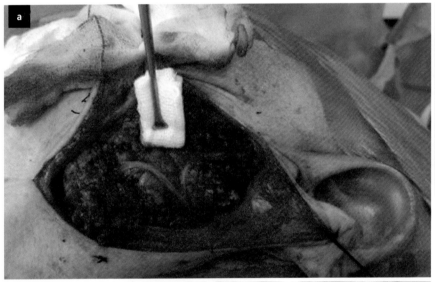
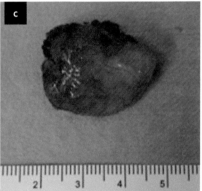
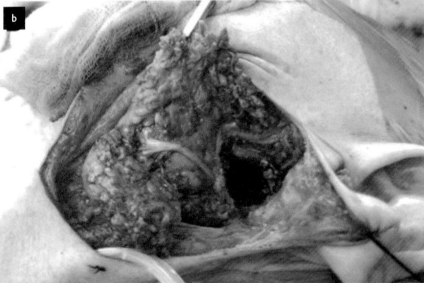

Figure 13-15. Partial mobilization of the facial nerve branches. If the tumor is located in one direction (a), all branches of the facial nerve should not be identified. Only affected branch is freed and the tumor is easily removed with gentle dissection (b and c).

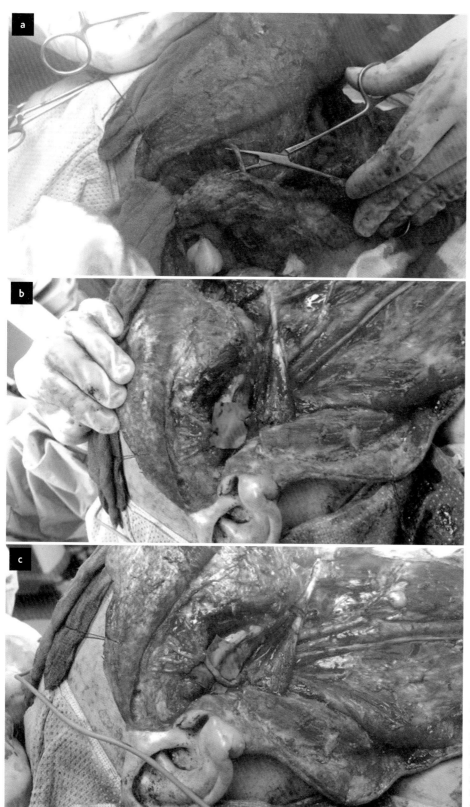

Figure 13-16. Reanimation of the facial nerve. If the facial nerve could not be identified due to the tumor invasion (a), the branches could be dissected (b) and reanimated. The sural nerve and the greater auricular nerve are often used as the interpositional graft (c).

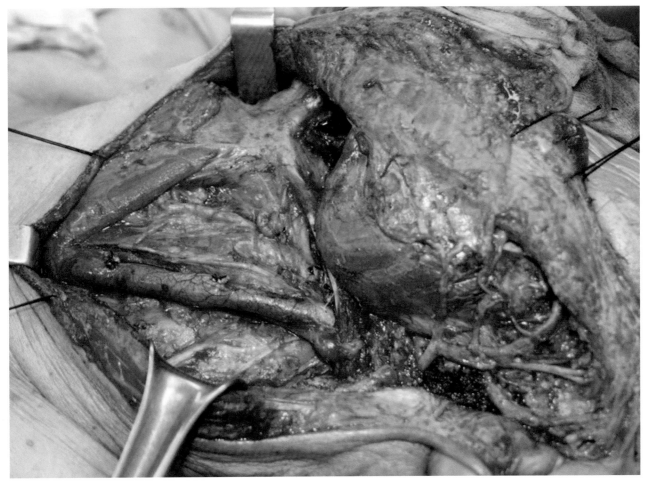

Figure 13-17. The transcervical-transparotid approach.

prestyloid parapharyngeal space component of the tumor. The entire tumor specimen can then be removed through the neck (**Figure 13-17**). Once the tumor is completely removed and bleeding is controlled, one drain is left in the parapharyngeal and the parotid space together. Wound closure is performed in the standard layered fashion.

7. Transmandibular approach

The transcervical approach to the parapharyngeal space with mandibulotomy provides better access.[9] Transmandibular approach are considered to manage

malignant tumors that invade skull base and its adjacent structures or for truly extensive and large benign tumors.[10,11]

Skin incision is done as mentioned above. After skin flap elevation, submandibular sialadenectomy could be carried out. The mandibular gingiva is sharply incised at the midline and elevated on a subperiosteal plane. A mandibulotomy is performed using the reciprocating saw first and the fine osteotome for last cutting. There are two different mandibulotomy approaches; Medial mandibulotomy anterior to mental foramen and lateral mandibulotomy posterior to

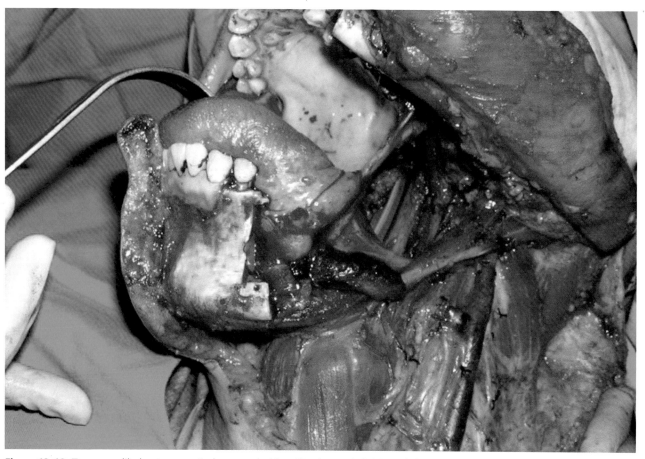

Figure 13-18. Transmandibular-transcervical approach. Identification and division of the stylomandibular ligament and the digastric muscles allows for dislocation of the mandible anteriorly to gain wider access to the parapharyngeal space. After swing of the mandible, the high cervical space is exposed.

mental foramen. Recently lateral mandibulotomy is seldom used because of its high morbidities including injury of the mental nerve and the mental artery. A lateral mandibulotomy site is almost included in the field of radiation therapy. The combination of radiation effect and loss of blood supply by dividing the mental artery in lateral mandibulotomy may result in the nonunion or osteo-radionecrosis of the mandible.[12] Medial mandibulotomy can be further classified into midline and paramidline mandibulotomy. Paramidline mandibulotomy, between the mandibular lateral incisor and canine, preserves the geniohyoid

and genioglossus muscles and appears to be a more versatile and preferable approach than midline mandibulotomy (**Figure 13-18**).[12]

The muscles of the mouth floor are sharply dissected from the mandible and the mandible is swung laterally to obtain the widest exposure of the PPS (**Figure 13-18**). After swinging the mandible neurovascular structures are followed from the neck to the skull base. A mandibulotomy site is fixed with two titanium miniplates. The mucosa incision is closed in layers with absorbable sutures. A suction drain is inserted in the neck field after thorough bleeding control.

IV. Summary

1. The parapharyngeal space (PPS) is a triangular compartment of the suprahyoid neck, lateral to the pharynx.
2. The PPS is divided by the styloid process along with the attaching muscles and tensor veli palatini fascia into a prestyloid and poststyloid compartment.
3. The prestyloid space contains the deep parotid lobe and minor salivary glands.
4. The poststyloid space contains the cranial nerves (IX, X, XI and XII), the critical vasculatures (the internal jugular vein, the internal carotid artery), the cervical sympathetic chain, and lymph nodes.
5. Tumors of the PPS account for 0.5-1.5% of all head and neck tumors. Approximately, 80% of these neoplasms are benign. Prestyloid tumors are commonly from salivary origin, while the poststyloid space is most often affected by neurogenic tumors.
6. Surgical approach should be selected according to the location of the tumor and its pathological entity.
7. The cervical and the transcervical-transparotid approach are widely used for surgical access. Under certain circumstances the transcervical-transmandibular and combined transoral approach may be used.

REFERENCES

1. van Hees T, van Weert S, Witte B, René Leemans C. Tumors of the parapharyngeal space: the VU University Medical Center experience over a 20-year period. Eur Arch Otorhinolaryngol 2018;275(4):967-72.

2. Stambuk HE, Patel SG. Imaging of the Parapharyngeal Space. Otolaryngol Clin North Am 2008;41:77-101.

3. Presutti L, Molteni G, Malvè L, Marchioni D, Ghidini A, Tassi S, et al. Parapharyngeal space tumors without mandibulotomy: our experience. Eur Arch Otorhinolaryngol 2012;269(1):265-73.

4. Mydlarz WK, Agrawal N. Transparotid and transcervical approaches for removal of deep lobe parotid gland and parapharyngeal space tumors. Oper Tech Otolayngol Head Neck Surg 2014;25(3):234-9.

5. Betka J, Chovanec M, Klozar J, Taudy M, Plzák J, Kodetová D, et al. Transoral and combined transoral-transcervical approach in the surgery of parapharyngeal tumors. Eur Arch Otorhinolaryngol 2010;267(5):765-72.

6. Panda S, Sikka K, Thakar A, Sharma SC, Krishnamurthy P. Transoral robotic surgery for the parapharyngeal space: expanding the transoral corridor. J Robot Surg 2020;14(1):61-7.

7. Chang SS, Goldenberg D, Koch WM. Transcervical approach to benign parapharyngeal space tumors. Ann Otol Rhinol Laryngol 2012;121(9):620-4.

8. Sun Y, Liu L, Han Y, Xu L, Zhang D, Wang H. The role of great auricular-facial nerve neurorrhaphy in facial nerve damage. Int J Clin Exp Med 2015;8(8):12970-6.

9. Abdel-Haleem A, El Sayed A, Hakeem HA. Transmandibular approach in parapharyngeal tumors: When to do it? Egypt J Ear Nose Throat Allied Sci 2011;12(1):25-31.

10. Luna-Ortiz K, Villa-Zepeda O, Carrillo JF, Molina-Frias E, Gómez-Pedraza A. Parapharyngeal space tumor: Submandibular approach without mandibulotomy. J Maxillofac Oral Surg 2018;17(4):616-24.

11. Basaran B, Polat B, Unsaler S, Ulusan M, Aslan I, Hafiz G. Parapharyngeal space tumours: the efficiency of a transcervical approach without mandibulotomy through review of 44 cases. Acta Otorhinolaryngol Ital 2014;34(5):310-6.

12. Pan W-L, Hao S-P, Lin Y-S, Chang K-P, Su J-L. The anatomical basis for mandibulotomy: midline versus paramidline. Laryngoscope 2003;113(2):377-80.

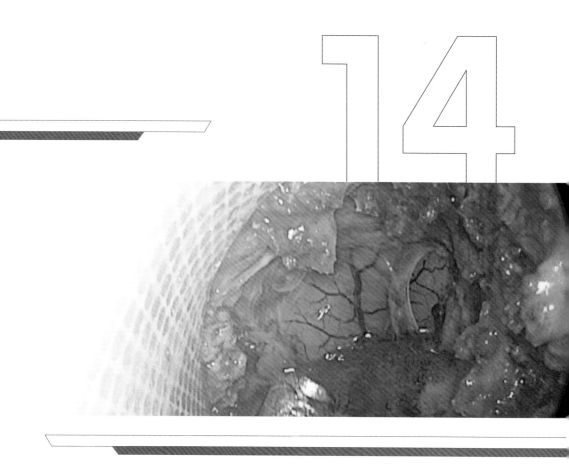

14

TRANS-ORBITAL APPROACH – SPHENO-ORBITAL MENINGIOMA

Min Ho Lee M.D., Ph.D., Doo-Sik Kong M.D., Ph.D.

I. Introduction

Spheno-orbital meningioma (SOM) arises from the sphenoid wing with or without intra-orbital extension and hyperostosis of the sphenoid bone.[1,2] SOM represents 9% of intracranial meningiomas. SOM can extend to evolve in an en plaque fashion or globulous type, and evokes hyperostosis in adjacent bony structures.[3,4] Hyperostosis of surrounding bones caused by SOM results in the direct compression of surrounding structures. Therefore, patients often visit clinics for proptosis, diplopia, and visual impairment, etc. (Figure 14-1).[5,6] As far, surgical approach of SOM has been assessed by transcranial approach, with pterional, or fronto-temporal craniotomy. But, it sometimes requires excessive retraction of the temporalis muscle followed by a zygomatic osteotomy. The goal of treatment for meningioma is achievement of gross total resection. In principle, it is impossible to remove tumors with Simpson grade 1 via the conventional trans-cranial approach.[2,7] Surgery of meningioma should be performed with the goal of achieving maximal safe resection.[8] Recently, endoscopic trans-orbital approach (eTOA) with a superior eyelid incision has been introduced as a minimally invasive technique.[9-12] Since it is possible to remove the involved bone and dura, Simpson grade 1 is theoretically possible. Furthermore, it leaves no definite skull base defect, and significant atrophy of the temporalis muscle, which results in cosmetic problem.[11-14] In this chapter the methods of eTOA are described with figures step-by-step. Figures in this chapter are included from several other cases to help readers' understanding.

1. Procedure

(1) Opening

Surgical procedures about eTOA were described in previous studies.[6,9,10,12,14-17] The patient is placed in a supine position in rigid 3-point fixation under general anesthesia.

After the neuro-navigation system is applied, a skin incision is made at the lateral half of the eyelid crease line for patients with an eyelid crease. The line is ex-

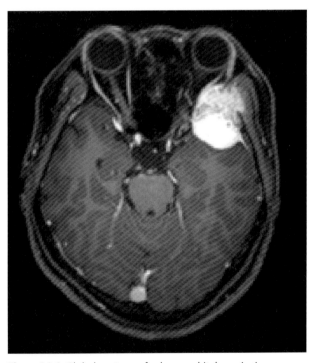

Figure 14-1. Globulous type of spheno-orbital meningioma.

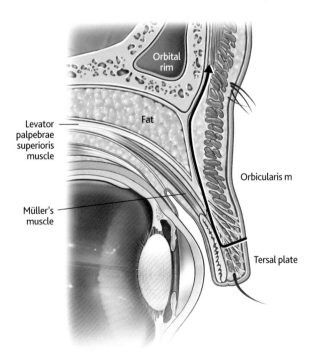

Figure 14-2. Illustration of superior eyelid skin incision.

tended about 1 cm laterally over the lateral orbital rim (**Figure 14-2**). The skin and orbicularis muscle flap are raised and extended superolaterally until the lateral orbital rim was reached. A periosteal incision is made on the lateral orbital rim after blunt dissection to the periosteum. The periosteum is elevated with a periosteal elevator (**Figure 14-3**). The dissection is extended to the superior and inferior orbital fissures with care to prevent orbital fat herniation. When more space should be needed, the lateral orbital rim is cut 5 mm superior to the fronto-zygomatic suture line and superior to the zygomatic arch line with a wire passer. The lateral orbital rim is resected using an osteotome and mallet (**Figure 14-4**).

(2) Craniectomy and tumor removal

A 0 degree rod-lens endoscope is introduced into the subperiosteal space, with the periorbita protected with a silastic sheet. A silastic sheet allows prevention of engorged orbital fat tissue as well as injury of periorbita. A periorbita is gently retracted with a suction tip, not with a fixed retractor. At an initial phase, a hand-held retraction of the orbit may be helpful to visualize inner anatomy. However, as gradual removal of the greater sphenoid wing is progressed, a wider surgical field can be obtained, resulting in the unnecessary hand-held retraction. After confirming the boundary of the tumor by neuro-navigation system, bony removal can be performed. When hyperostotic sphenoid bone is removed gradually, frontal dura and temporal dura can be identified (**Figure 14-5**). Tumor removal proceeds in the same way as other transcranial surgery. After internal tumor debulking is performed using an ultrasonic aspirator and the margin is secured, sharp dissection from brain parenchyma is performed to remove it (**Figure 14-6**).

(3) Closing

After the tumor removal, harvested abdominal fat can be grafted to fill the dead space intra-durally. Allogenic dermis or autologous fascia lata would be grafted on the dura as in-lay and out-lay with bilayer button (**Figure 14-7**).[11,18] Artificial bone plate is placed to cover the craniectomy site and prevents enophthalmos. The orbital rim is repositioned. The periosteum, subcutaneous tissue, and skin are sutured layer by layer.

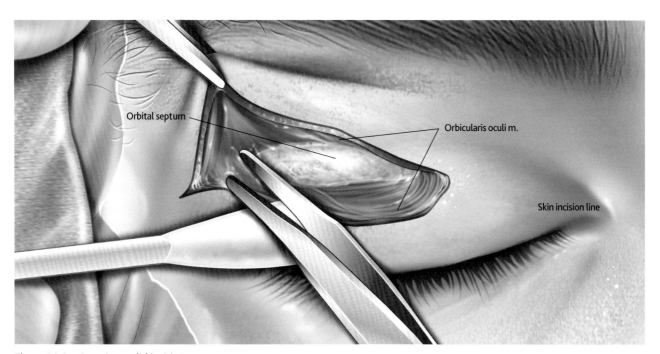

Figure 14-3a. Superior eyelid incision.

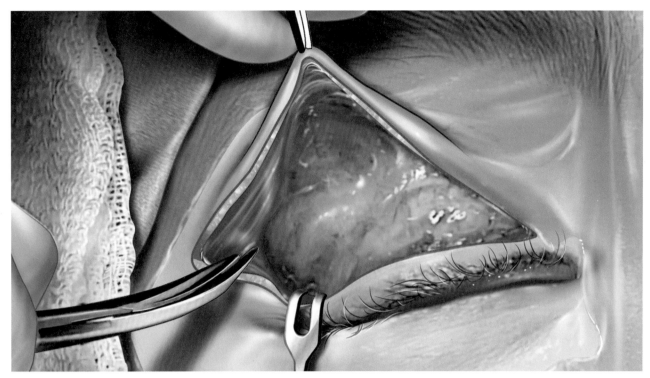

Figure 14-3b. Superior eyelid crease incision with raised orbicularis muscle flap.

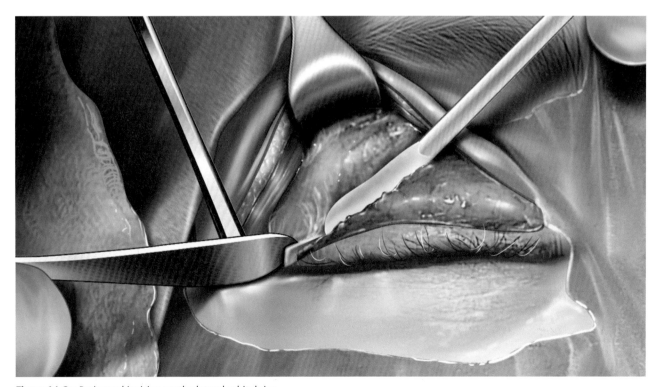

Figure 14-3c. Periosteal incision on the lateral orbital rim

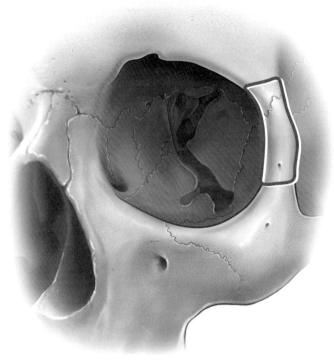

Figure 14-4. Illustration of the lateral orbital rim to be removed

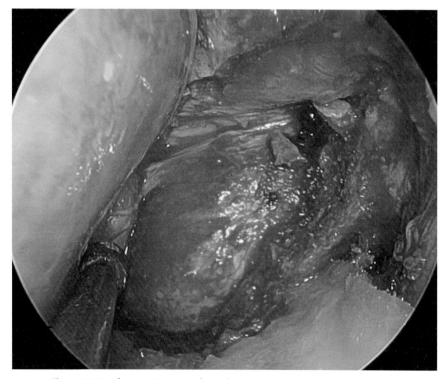

Figure 14-5. After craniectomy, frontal and temporal dura can be identified.

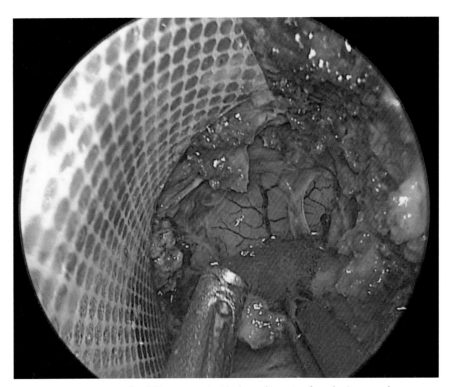

Figure 14-6. Tumor should be removed with sharp dissection from brain parenchyma.

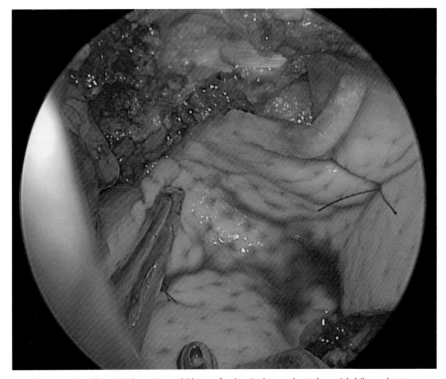

Figure 14-7. Allogenic dermis would be grafted as in-lay and out-lay with bilayer button.

II. Tip and summary

As eTOA is an unfamiliar approach to neurosurgeons and ENT surgeons., it is very important to have sufficient prior knowledge about orbital anatomy. Since the initial surgical field is narrow compared to the endonasal approach, it is essential to secure the space by drilling the greater sphenoid wing comprising the lateral orbital wall. A lateral orbital rim osteotomy can contribute to the improvement of the gross total resection rate.[6] If lumbar drainage is performed in advance and the intracranial pressure is lowered, the operation may be much easier. To avoid cosmetic complications, collaboration with a plastic surgeon or ophthalmic surgeon can help improve the outcome of the surgery.

The eTOA may still be in its infancy, but it is an approach that has a very high potential in the future, showing a versatile possibility. It is considered to be a very effective approach to surgery for SOM.

REFERENCES

1.   Terrier L-M, et al. Spheno-orbital meningiomas surgery: Multicenter management study for complex extensive tumors. World Neurosurg 2018;112:e145-56.

2.   Bikmaz, K., R. Mrak, and O.J.J.o.n. Al-Mefty. Management of bone-invasive, hyperostotic sphenoid wing meningiomas. J Neurosurg 2007;107(5):905-12.

3.   Amirjamshidi A, Abbasioun K, Amiri RS, Ardalan A, Hashemi SMR. Lateral orbitotomy approach for removing hyperostosing en plaque sphenoid wing meningiomas. Description of surgical strategy and analysis of findings in a series of 88 patients with long-term follow up. Surg Neurol Int 2015;6(1):79.

4.   Samadian M, Sharifi G, Mousavinejad SA, Amin AA, Ebrahimzadeh K, Tavassol HH, et al. Surgical outcomes of sphenoorbital en plaque meningioma: A 10-year experience in 57 consecutive cases. World Neurosurg 2020;144:e576-81.

5.   Dallan, I., et al. Endoscopic Transorbital Superior Eyelid Approach for the Management of Selected Spheno-orbital Meningiomas: Preliminary Experience. Operative Neurosurgery 2017;14(3):243-51.

6.   Kong D.S., Y.H. Kim, and C.K. Hong. Optimal indications and limitations of endoscopic transorbital superior eyelid surgery for spheno-orbital meningiomas. J Neurosurg 2020;134(5):1472-9.

7.   Simpson D. The recurrence of intracranial meningiomas after surgical treatment. J Neurol Neurosurg Psychiatry 1957;20(1):22-39.

8.   Schwartz T.H., McDermott M.W. The Simpson grade: abandon the scale but preserve the message. J Neurosurg 2020;1-8.

9.   Dallan I, et al. Endoscopic transorbital superior eyelid approach for the management of selected spheno-orbital meningiomas: Preliminary experience. Oper Neurosurg (Hagerstown) 2018;14(3):243-51.

10.   Di Somma A, Andaluz N, Cavallo LM, de Notaris M, Dallan I, Solari D, et al. Endoscopic transorbital superior eyelid approach: anatomical study from a neurosurgical perspective. J Neurosurg 2018;129(5):1203-16.

11.   Kong D.S., Young SM, Hong C-K, Kim Y-D, Hong SD, Choi JW, et al. Clinical and ophthalmological outcome of endoscopic transorbital surgery for cranioorbital tumors. J Neurosurg 2018;131(3):667-75.

12.   Lee M.H., et al. Endoscopic endonasal versus transorbital surgery for middle cranial Fossa tumors: Comparison of clinical outcomes based on surgical corridors. World Neurosurg 2019;122:e1491-504.

13.   Jeon C, et al. Endoscopic transorbital surgery for Meckel's cave and middle cranial fossa tumors: surgical technique and early results. J Neurosurg 2018;131(4):1-10.

14.   Park H.H., et al. Endoscopic transorbital and endonasal approach for trigeminal schwannomas: a retrospective multicenter analysis (KOSEN-005). J Neurosurg 2020;133(2):467-76.

15.   Locatelli D., et al. Transorbital endoscopic approaches to the skull base: current concepts and future perspectives. J Neurosurg Sci 2016;60(4):514-25.

16.   Park H.H., et al. Comparative analysis of endoscopic transorbital approach and extended mini-pterional approach for sphenoid wing meningiomas with osseous involvement: Preliminary surgical results. World Neurosurg 2020;139:e1-12.

17.   In Woo K, et al. Orbital decompressive effect of endoscopic transorbital surgery for sphenoorbital meningioma. Arbeitsphysiologie 2021;259(4):1015-24.

18.   Luginbuhl AJ, Campbell PG, Evans J, Rosen M. Endoscopic repair of high-flow cranial base defects using a bilayer button. Laryngoscope 2010;120(5):876-80.

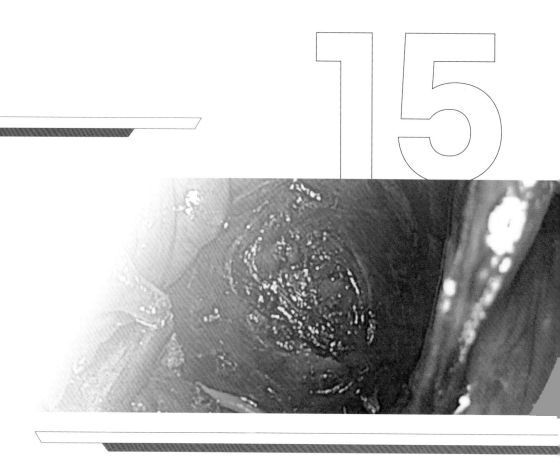

ENDOSCOPIC TRANSORBITAL APPROACH FOR ORBITAL TUMOR

Kyung Hwan Kim M.D., Ph.D., Doo-Sik Kong M.D., Ph.D.

I. Introduction

Endoscopic transorbital surgery has been adopted with increasing frequency over the last decade. While initially limited to the surgical management of pathologies involving orbit, endoscopic transorbital approach is now allowing to resect a wide range of skull base lesions.[1] The endoscopic transorbital approaches are indicated for the treatment of pathologies located within or adjacent to the orbit, and can be combined with transnasal, transmaxillary, or supraorbital paths.[2] Operating through the orbits might reduce hospitalization time and disfiguring after transfacial/transcranial surgery, and overcome limitations of endoscopic transnasal surgery such as visualization of certain structures and limited working angle.[3] In the literature, the endoscopic transorbital approaches to the orbit and skull base are based on 4 pillar approaches through orbital quadrants: superior eyelid crease, precaruncular, lateral retrocanthal, and preseptal lower eyelid which cross the superior, medial, lateral, and inferior orbital quadrants, respectively.[3] The superior eyelid crease approach, also named as upper eyelid approach, is the most common route to reach the superior orbit, frontal sinus, inferior portion of anterior cranial fossa, anterior skull base, and middle cranial fossa.1 The precaruncular approach provides a direct and avascular access to medial orbital roof, lamina papyracea, ethmoidal arteries, optic nerve, and the central corridor towards the anterior skull base.[4] The lateral retrocanthal approach enables to access to the deep lateral orbit, infratemporal and temporal fossa. The preseptal approach is useful to access to the inferior orbit and can be combined with lateral retrocanthal or precaruncular approaches to expose the orbit widely. Here we describe two representative approaches, superior eyelid crease and precaruncular approaches.

Before surgery, a complete neuro-radiological routine study, including brain and orbital CT and MRI scans, and a thorough ophthalmologic examination are inevitable for success of the surgery.

II. Procedure

The patient is placed supine with the head in slight flexion and fixed by a 3-pin Mayfield head holder. Surgical skin and conjunctiva preparation with low concentration povidone solution (5%) is made followed by aseptic surgical draping. We recommend exposing both eyes after draping and the use of a lubricated corneal protector to check size of both pupils during surgery.

1. Superior eyelid crease approach

Skin incision is made along the crease of the upper eyelid. Dissection is continued through the orbicularis oculi muscle, and a skin-muscle flap is raised superiorly and laterally until the identification of the orbital rim (**Figure 15-1**). The dissection is carried out in a preseptal plane and care must be taken not to dissect into the fat pad deep to the orbital septum and the levator aponeurosis. Once the orbital rim is reached, the periosteum is incised by a fine monopolar coagulator, and blunt dissection of the periorbital in a cranio-caudal and latero-medial fashion through the orbital roof and lateral wall (**Figure 15-2**). Since the orbital structures are free from their supero-lateral attachments, a hand-held retractor is gently set in place in an inferomedial fashion, and the endoscope is brought to the

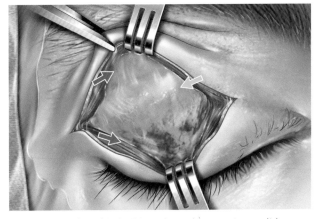

Figure 15-1. After skin incision along the superior eyelid crease (right eye) and dissection through the orbicularis oculi (blue arrow), orbital septum (yellow arrow) is exposed.

field. The lacrimal foramen (cranio-orbital foramen), which transmits the recurrent meningeal branch of the lacrimal artery, is a good landmark for the sub-periosteal dissection and is presented in 50 to 60% of patients (**Figure 15-3**). It is located 1 to 2 cm anterior to the superior orbital fissure along the superior edge of the lateral wall. After sacrificing recurrent meningeal branch, further dissection to the edge of superior and inferior orbital fissure is made. In most cases, identification of the superior orbital fissure is paramount to achieve adequate orientation.

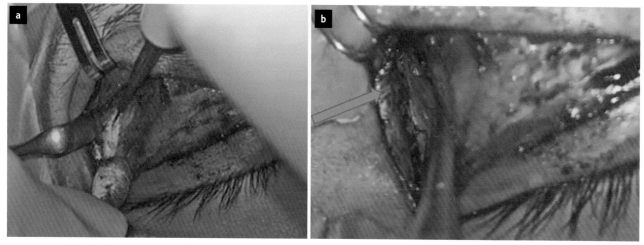

Figure 15-2. (a) orbital rim is identified and periosteum is incised with monopolar coagulator; (b) periorbita is separated from the orbital rim (blue arrow) and the lateral orbital wall using a blunt dissector

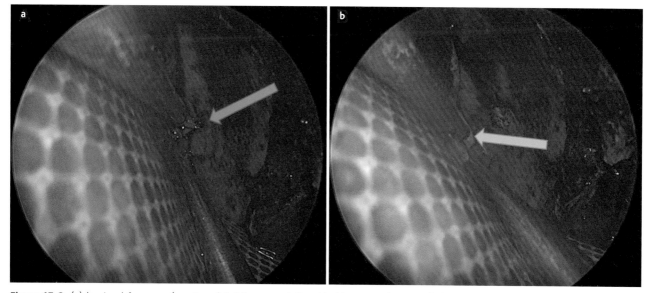

Figure 15-3. (a) lacrimal foramen (cranio-orbital foramen, left orbit, blue arrow), transmitting recurrent meningeal branch of lacrimal artery, is located before reaching the superior orbital fissure; (b) the lateral edge of superior orbital fissure (yellow arrow) is an important landmark of endoscopic transorbital approach

2. Precaruncular approach

This approach provides a direct, avascular approach to the medial region of the orbit and heals rapidly without scarring (**Figure 15-4**). The incision is begun at the conjunctiva between the caruncle and skin (medial to the caruncle) with a fine scissors or a sharp monopolar tip (**Figure 15-5**). It is extended superiorly and inferiorly, following the avascular plane of superior and inferior limbs of the posterior limb of the medial canthal tendon. The periosteum is incised immediately posterior to crista laminalis (the posterior border of the lacrimal fossa). The periorbital is then lifted laterally off the medial orbital wall (lamina papyracea) with a periosteal elevator until the anterior ethmoidal artery is encountered. The level of the anterior skull base can be estimated by the ethmoidal bundles which are found along the fronto-ethmoidal suture. Anterior ethmoidal arteries can be cauterized and transected. Then, an endoscope is introduced and continues the subperiosteal dissection from the floor to roof. The posterior ethmoidal artery is then identified and it warns the surgeon that the optic nerve is close (around 7 mm). The dissection continues posteriorly until the optic nerve is identified. The optic nerve is located at the posterior aspect of the medial orbit, in the same plane as the ethmoidal arteries.

3. Identifying and resecting orbital tumor

During the subperiosteal dissection, placing a Silastic sheet and a handheld, malleable retractor over the periorbita is recommended to protect and to retract gently the orbit. We perform a surgical approach by two surgeons with the aid of a self-retaining pneumatic endoscope holder. If needed, additional craniectomy takes place first depending on the pathology. After a neuronavigation check, the periorbital overlying the lesion or the tumor capsule is sharply opened, and the tumor was carefully removed (**Figure 15-6**). General principle of tumor resection is the same as other neurological surgeries.

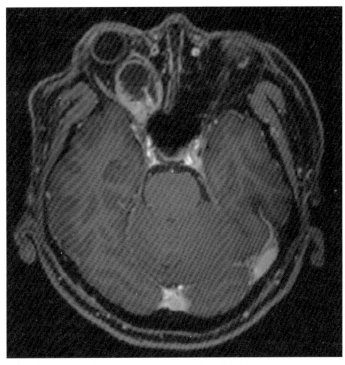

Figure 15-4. The patient presented with right visual dimness and proptosis and MRI scan shows a large cystic mass with heterogeneous T1-enhancement is located in the medial portion of the right orbit; the patient underwent an endoscopic transorbital surgery via a precaruncular approach.

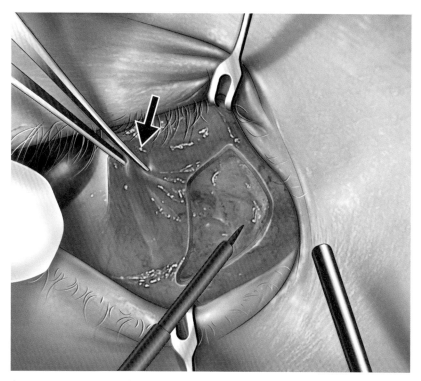

Figure 15-5. A conjunctival incision is performed between caruncle (blue arrow) and skin

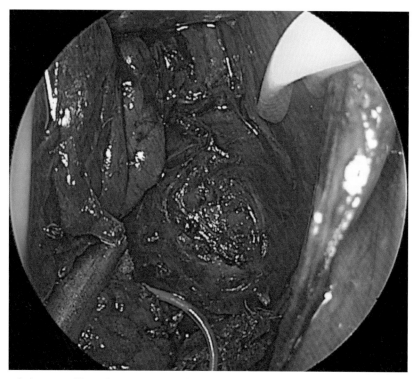

Figure 15-6. Tumor capsule is exposed in endoscopic view and incised for internal debulking; yellow rubber band marks medial rectus.

4. Reconstruction

In cases in which the dura mater is opened and/or CSF leakage is evident, skull base reconstruction using a multilayer fashion including dural substitute and button grafts composed of a bilayer of autologous fascia lata or acellular dermal matrix allograft. A wedge-shaped porous polyethylene can be introduced as a rigid buttress to prevent enophthalmos when a large bony defect is expected. The orbital periosteum and the skin or conjunctival incision is closed layer by layer.

III. Tip and summary

First of all, multidisciplinary team discussions involving neurosurgeons, ENT and ophthalmic surgeons are essential to plan surgical strategies and to manage patients. Recently, Jeon et al. proposed a four-zone model based on the location of the tumor epicenter around the optic nerve in the coronal plane to select optimal endoscopic transorbital and/or transnasal approaches for orbital tumors.[5] Selecting an appropriate combinative approach can improve surgical outcome and reduce morbidity.

Second, in case of orbital fat exiting from the orbital structures, silicon pads can be used under the retractor to maximize control. We recommend using a hand-held, dynamic retraction rather than fixed compression of the orbital structures to avoid direct or vascular related orbital damage.

The endoscopic transorbital approach provides substantial advantages in treating orbital tumors. It allows the surgeon to avoid a large craniotomy and extra soft tissue dissection and provides a relatively short and direct corridor. This versatile approach is extremely useful and an important supplement to the conventional skull base approaches that should be in the arming of a skull base team.

REFERENCES

1. Vural A, Carobbio ALC, Ferrari M, Rampinelli V, Schreiber A, Mattavelli D, et al. Transorbital endoscopic approaches to the skull base: a systematic literature review and anatomical description. Neurosurg Rev 2021;44(5):2857-78.

2. Balakrishnan K, Moe KS. Applications and outcomes of orbital and transorbital endoscopic surgery. Otolaryngol Head Neck Surg 2011; 144(5):815-20.

3. Moe KS, Bergeron CM, Ellenbogen RG. Transorbital neuroendoscopic surgery. Neurosurgery 2010;67(3 Suppl Operative):ons16-28.

4. Raza SM, Quinones-Hinojosa A, Lim M, Boahene KDO. The transconjunctival transorbital approach: a keyhole approach to the midline anterior skull base. World Neurosurg 2013;80(6):864-71.

5. Jeon C, Hong SD, Woo KI, Seol HJ, Nam DH, Lee JI, et al. Use of endoscopic transorbital and endonasal approaches for 360 degrees circumferential access to orbital tumors. J Neurosurg 2020;1-10.

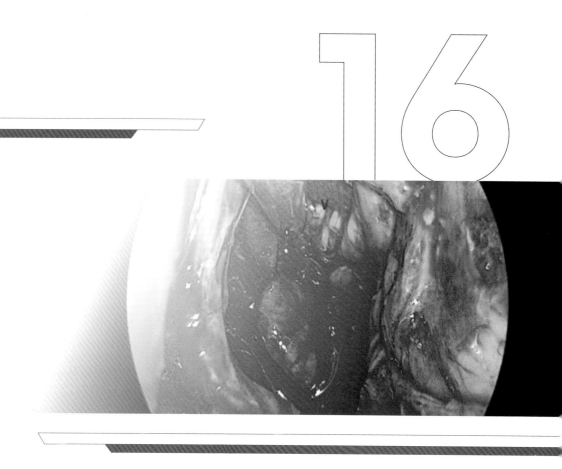

16

ENDOSCOPIC TRANSORBITAL APPROACH TO THE CAVERNOUS SINUS

Chang-Ki Hong M.D., Ph.D.

I. Introduction

Traditional open craniotomy to the cavernous sinus (CS) have been extensively described with wide-ranging outcomes in terms of morbidity and mortality. Classic transcranial approaches to CS require extensive removal of bone and muscles and excessive brain retraction. Although each approach has its own benefits and limitations, all methods commonly require brain retraction to some extent and even warrant extensive bone removal, including removal of zygomatic bone and the squamous part of the temporal bone for wide exposure. Surgical approaches to the skull base (SB) significantly evolved over the last decades.

Recent reports have studied endoscopic approaches to the lateral cavernous sinus facilitated via supraorbital craniotomy or via transorbital approaches that provide surgical access to the CS and adjacent skull base. The endoscopic transorbital approach (eTOA) is a more effective and targeted approach to disease of the anterior cranial fossa. In addition to the visualization of middle cranial fossa tumors, a surgical corridor through this approach allows excellent visualization of the lateral cavernous sinus while avoiding the need for brain retraction.

II. Surgical techniques

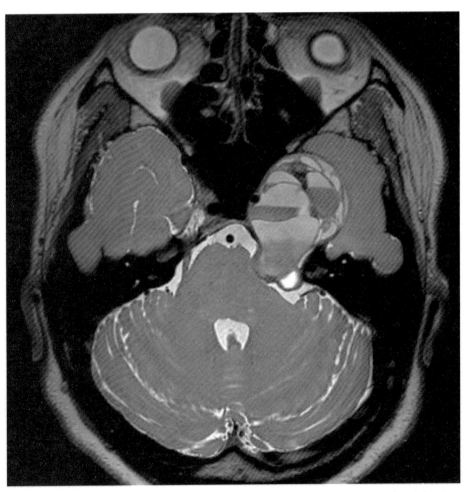

Figure 16-1. A 38-year-old woman with trigeminal schwannoma involving the Meckel's cave presented with facial numbness. Preoperative proton density MR image indicated that the tumor involved the cavernous sinus and extended into the posterior fossa.

III. Position and eyelid phase

The patient was placed in a supine position with the head in a neutral or slight flexion position. Having the head in a flexion position affords easy surgical access to the floor of the temporal lobe.

The skin incision was performed in the natural eyelid crease, extending from the lateral canthus to approximately 1.5 to 2 cm medially (**Figure 16-2**). A corneal protector may be used.

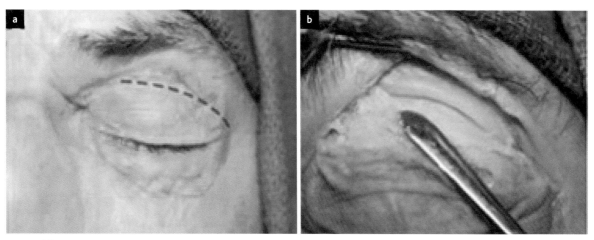

Figure 16-2. (a) Incision along the superior eyelid crease. Dissection of connective tissue from the orbital rim exposing the periosteum of the left orbit. (b) the periosteum was incised at the orbital rim, over the frontal bone. Subsequently, the periosteum is dissected inferiorly around the orbital rim, preserving the periorbita to protect the orbital contents and prevent orbital fat herniation.

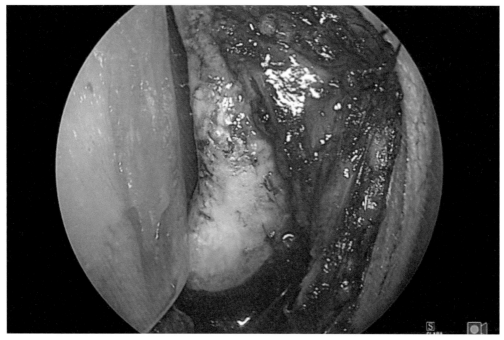

Figure 16-3. The entire globe and periorbital are gently retracted medially with a malleable brain retractor. Endoscopic view of the initial peeling of the orbital septum away from the orbital wall.

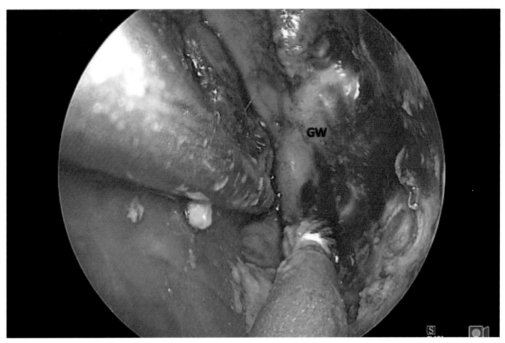

Figure 16-4. The eTOA is performed using a rigid endoscope 4 mm in diameter, 18 cm in length, with a 0 and 30° lens (Karl Storz, Tuttlingen, Germany). It has to be stressed that angled endoscopes were very useful during the drilling of the greater wing of the sphenoid bone. Once periosteal dissection along the superolateral orbital wall exposed the lateral margin of the SOF, the greater wing of the sphenoid was then removed until the dura mater covering the temporal pole came into view.

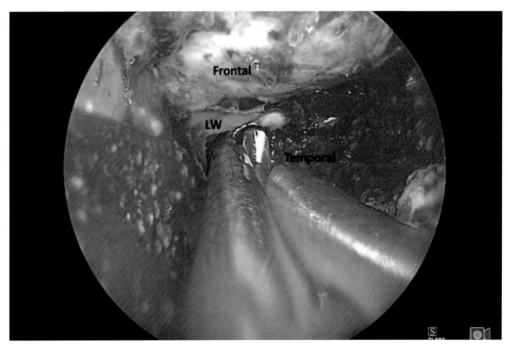

Figure 16-5. Sphenoid ridge is removed with pituitary rongeurs after drilling; removal of this sliver of bone facilitates peeling of meningo-orbital band (MOB).

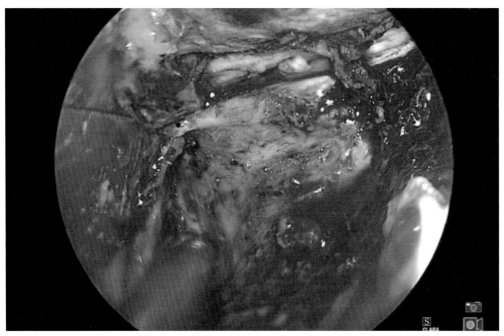

Figure 16-6. *, MOB. At this phase, the first landmark was the MOB. The MOB is a sagittally oriented structure between the temporo-basal dura and the lateral aspect of the periorbita. The MOB runs along the lateral border of the superior orbital fissure (SOF). It is typically exposed transcranially via a frontotemporal craniotomy along the lateral border of the SOF when the temporal basal dura is fully retracted. From an anatomical viewpoint the MOB has been described as leading directly to the interdural space of the cavernous sinus.

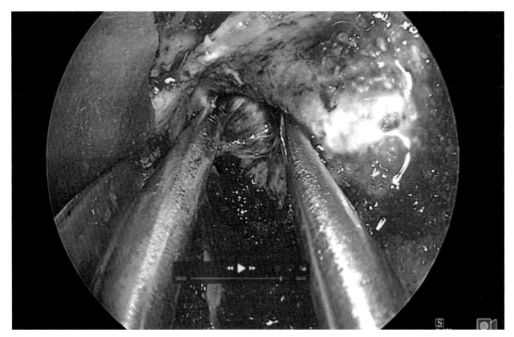

Figure 16-7. A cutting and gentle dissection of MOB "naturally" reveals the lateral wall of the cavernous sinus via an interdural pathway. It offers access to the inner layer of the lateral wall without the need to enter the venous compartment of the sinus itself, and, even more importantly, it provides access without manipulation of the CS' cranial nerves. The lateral wall of the cavernous sinus is formed by two dural layers: a thin inner layer, the periosteal dura, containing the III, IV and V cranial nerve on their way to the SOF; and an outer layer, the meningeal dura, which is thicker with a pearly grey color.

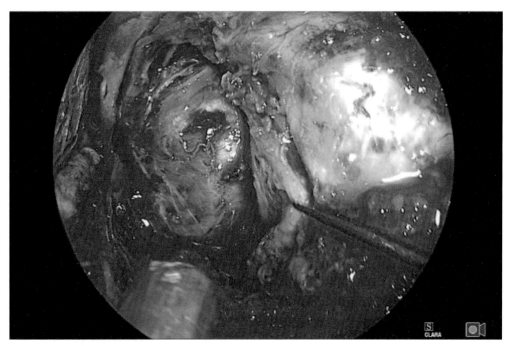

Figure 16-8. At the lower lateral edge of the cavernous sinus the two layers usually divide, with the meningeal layer and the outer part of the periosteal layer extending upward to form the lateral wall of the cavernous sinus, whereas the periosteal layer continues medially to form part of the medial sinus wall. Dissections on the lateral sinus wall reveal that the thicker outer layer (a continuation of the meningeal layer) peels away, leaving the thin inner layer (an extension of the periosteal layer) covering the nerves in the lateral wall. The two layers are only loosely attached, and it is easy to recognize a cleavage plane between them.

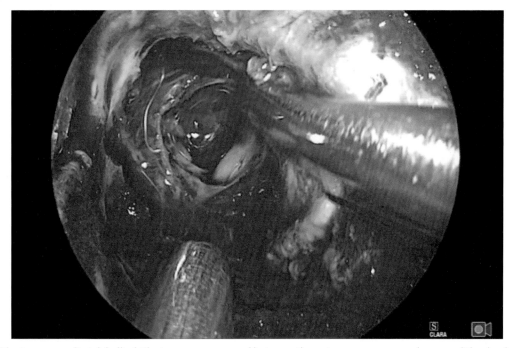

Figure 16-9. The tumor was first debulked. The tumor was exposed between the outer cavernous membrane and the dural propria. After removal of the tumor within Meckel's cave, some portion of the tumor extending into the posterior fossa was found.

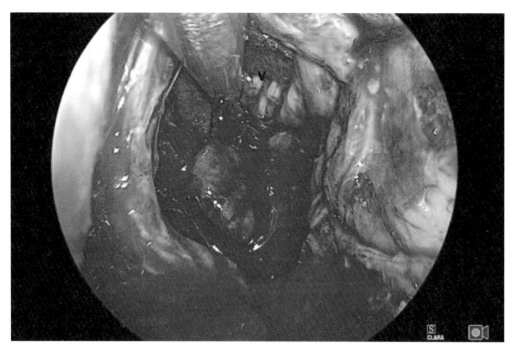

Figure 16-10. Trigeminal nerve was revealed after the tumor was totally removed.

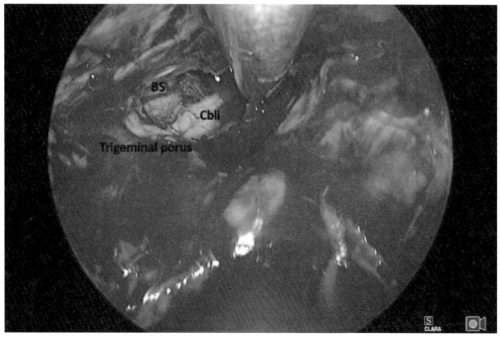

Figure 16-11. Brain stem and cerebellum was visualized through porus trigeminus.

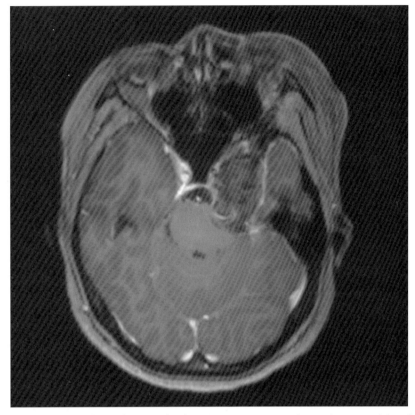

Figure 16-12. Postoperative gadolinium-enhanced T1-weighted MR images. Gross-total resection was achieved via transorbital corridor. The transorbital surgical corridor used to approach the lesion is visible.

REFERENCES

1. Dallan I, Castelnuovo P, Locatelli D, Turri-Zanoni M, AlQahtani A, Battaglia P, et al. Multiportal combined transorbital transnasal endoscopic approach for the management of selected skull base lesions: Preliminary experience. World Neurosurg 2015;84(1):97-107.

2. Dallan I, Castelnuovo P, Turri-Zanoni M, Fiacchini G, Locatelli D, Battaglia P, et al. Transorbital endoscopic assisted management of intraorbital lesions: lessons learned from our first 9 cases. Rhinology 2016;54(3):247-53.

3. Di Somma A, Andaluz N, Cavallo LM, Topczewski TE, Frio F, Gerardi RM, et al. Endoscopic transorbital route to the petrous apex: a feasibility anatomic study. Acta Neurochir (Wien) 2018;160(4):707-20.

4. Fukuda H, Evins AI, Burrell JC, Iwasaki K, Stieg PE, Bernardo A. The meningo-orbital band: Microsurgical anatomy and surgical detachment of the membranous structures through a frontotemporal craniotomy with removal of the anterior clinoid process. J Neurol Surg B Skull Base 2014;75(2):125-32.

5. Inoue T, Rhoton AL Jr, Theele D, Barry ME. Surgical approaches to the cavernous sinus: A microsurgical study. Neurosurgery 1990;26(6):903-32.

6. Jeon C, Hong CK, Woo KI, et al. Endoscopic transorbital surgery for Meckel's cave and middle cranial fossa tumors: surgical technique and early results. J Neurosurg 2019;131(4):1126-35.

7. Kong DS, Hong CK, Hong SD, et al. Selection of endoscopic or transcranial surgery for tuberculum sellae meningiomas according to specific anatomical features: a retrospective multicenter analysis (KOSEN-002). J Neurosurg 2018;130(3):838-47.

8. Locatelli D, Pozzi F, Turri-Zanoni M, Battaglia P, Santi L, Dallan I, et al. Transorbital endoscopic approaches to the skull base: current concepts and future perspectives. J Neurosurg Sci 2016;60:514-25.

9. Moe KS, Bergeron CM, Ellenbogen RG. Transorbital neuroendoscopic surgery. Neurosurgery 2010;67(3 Suppl Operative):ons16-28.

10. Park HH, Hong SD, Kim YH, et al. Endoscopic transorbital and endonasal approach for trigeminal schwannomas: a retrospective multicenter analysis (KOSEN-005). J Neurosurg 2020;133(2):467-76.

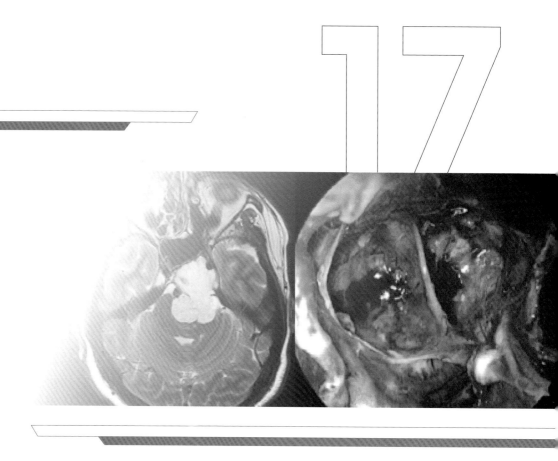

ENDOSCOPIC TRANS-CLIVAL AND PETROUS APPROACH

Yong Hwy Kim M.D., Ph.D.

I. Introduction

The clivus and ventral area to the brainstem is the most difficult zone to be accessed by the trans-cranial approach due to the midline, deep location and long vertical length. In addition, the paramedian locations of the cranial nerves posed the risk of damage during the surgical manipulation in these areas. Endoscopic trans-clival and -petrous approach provides direct access to the entire clivus and the adjacent medial petrous bone via nasal cavity without the manipulating or crossing the cranial nerves because there were no neurovascular structures passing the clivus.

The clivus, formed by the sphenoid and occipital bones, is a wide shallow depression, sloping anteriorly and upward from the foramen magnum. It is conventionally divided into 3 sections to facilitate the selection of a specific surgical approach.[1] The upper section of the clivus corresponds to the region of the dorsum sellae and posterior clinoid process. The middle section of the clivus is located between the Dorello's canal and the pars nervosa of the jugular foramen. The lower section of the clivus extends from the pars nervosa of the jugular foramen to the foramen magnum. The most adjacent cranial nerve to the clivus was CN VI passing the Dorello's canal and the paraclival internal carotid artery (ICA) bounded the clival recess and these two structures are the lateral limitation of endoscopic transclival approach. In cadaveric study, the distance between the midline and petro-sphenoidal foramen where the abducens nerve pass through was 10.5±1 mm and the distance from dorsum sellae to a line between bilateral petro-sphenoidal foramen was 16.5±1.5 mm.[2] This area is applicable to the upper clivus. The lateral limitations of the middle and lower section of clivus are foramen lacerum and hypoglossal canal.

II. Procedures

1. Nasoseptal flap

The design of nasoseptal flap was determined by the direction of septal deviation, distance to the skull base defect skull base defect and side to sacrifice the sphenopalatine artery to lateral extension. In general, the nasoseptal flap in the transclival and petrosal approaches should be larger and longer than that in the trans-tubercular approach, because the clivus is wider and deeper than tuberculum and sella. The bilateral nasoseptal flap is recommendable in cases of skull base defect larger than 2/3 of clivus. The flap should be prepared in the contralateral nasal cavity with the ipsilateral reverse flap , facilitating the flap harvest site healing and providing the wide surgical window in case requiring the trans-pterygoid approaches.

2. Procedures for the lateral approach

The resection of turbinates or ethmoidectomy are not necessary for the lesion limited between the bilateral paraclival ICA. The contralateral nasoseptal flap, resection of the ipsilateral middle turbinates, ipsilateral maxillary antrostomy, opening of the ipsilateral pterygopalatine fossa, ligation of the ipsilateral internal maxillary artery, and opening of the ipsilateral lateral recess of sphenoid are required for the trans-pterous approach for the lesion extending laterally to the paraclival ICA.

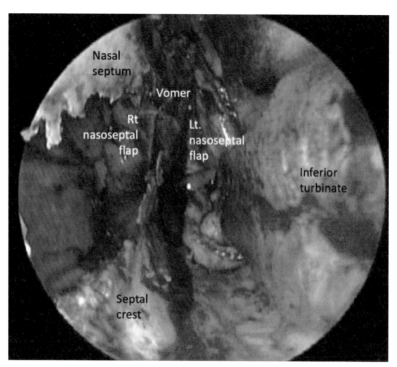

Figure 17-1a. Design of the bilateral nasoseptal flap. The nasal crest should be drilled out and flattened for the surgical freedom in the manipulation of lower clivus.

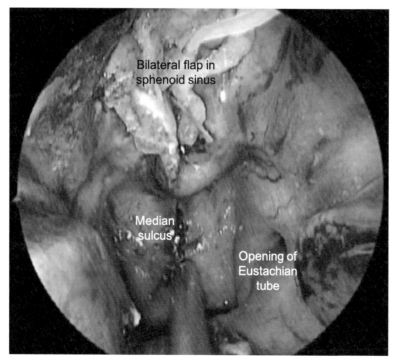

Figure 17-1b. Incision of median sulcus of nasopharynx to expose the lower clivus. The bilateral nasoseptal flaps are storage in the sphenoid sinus after sphenoidotomy

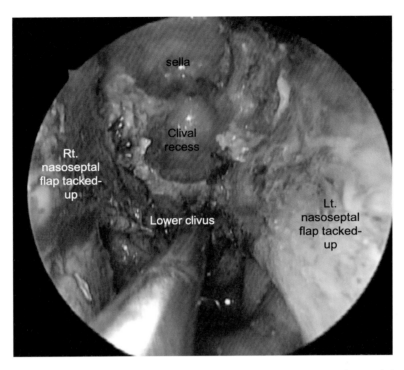

Figure 17-1c. Exposure of clivus. The anterior border of bilateral nasoseptal flaps are tacked-up and tracted through the each nostrils to secure the wide nasal cavity and basiopharyngeal fascia was dissected to expose the lower clivus.

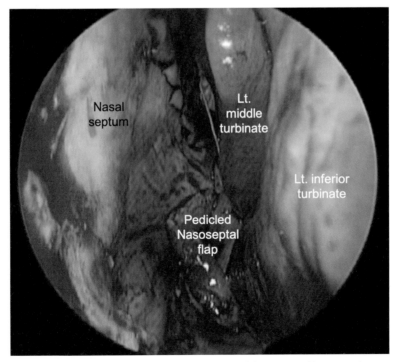

Figure 17-2a. Contralateral pedicle nasoseptal flap and the removed bony nasal septum.

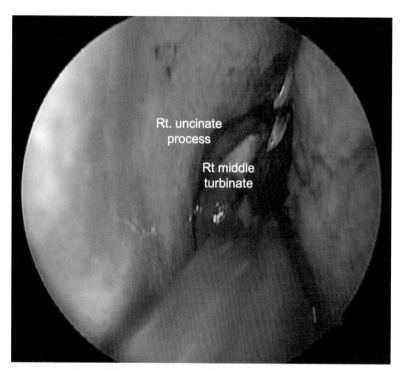

Figure 17-2b. Resection of ipsilateral middle turbinates.

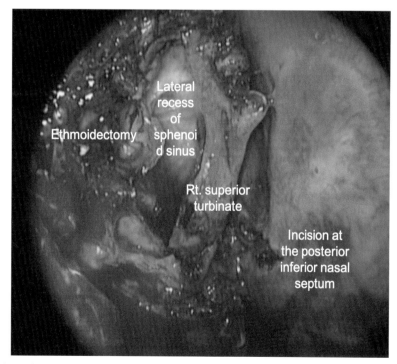

Figure 17-2c. Ipsilateral ethmoidectomy with the preservation of ipsilateral superior turbinate. The linear horizontal incision was made at the posterior inferior side of ipsilateral septal mucosa.

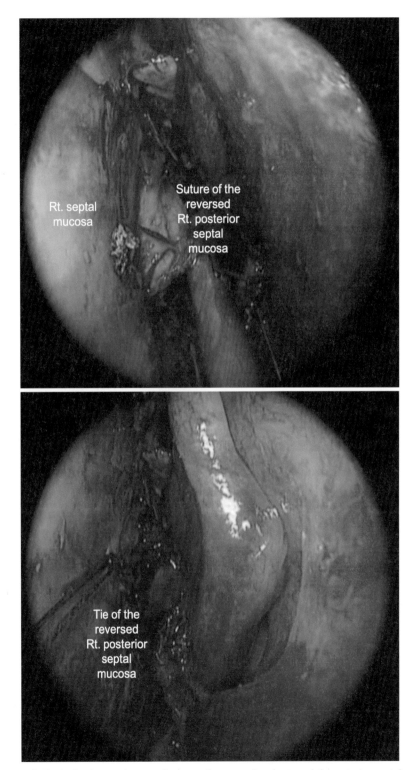

Figure 17-2d. The incised posterior septal mucosa is reversed and sutured the anterior septal mucosa.

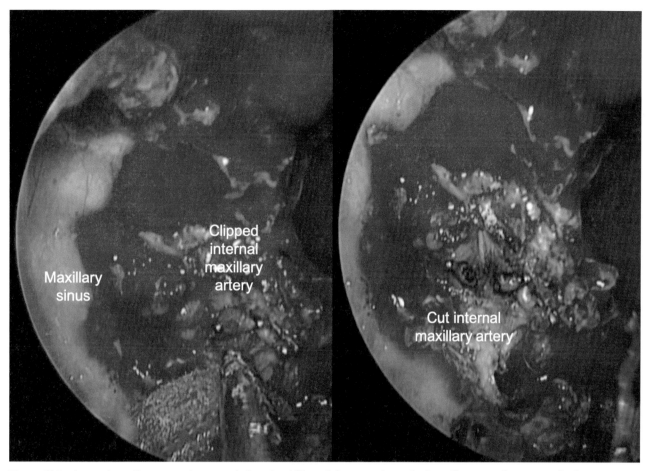

Figure 17-2e. Internal maxillary artery is exposed after the drilling of the posterior wall of maxillary sinus (anterior wall of pterygopalatine fossa) and dissection of fascia and fat of pterygopalatine fossa and then it was clipped and cut to expose the inferior side of the lateral recess of sphenoid sinus.

3. Skull base works

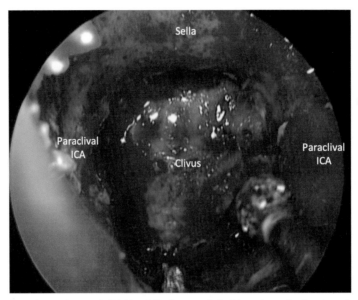

Figure 17-3a. All septations in the sphenoid sinus should be drilled out and skull base bone is also denuded for the surgical manipulation and engraft the skull base reconstruction materials including nasoseptal flap. The clivus was drilled out from the center at the lower margin of the required bony window and then expanded upward to secure the clear surgical field. Tailed bone drilling is performed in eggshell fashion. The venous bleeding from the basilar plexus is controlled with injectable hemostatic materials and bleeding from the bone marrow is done with bone wax.

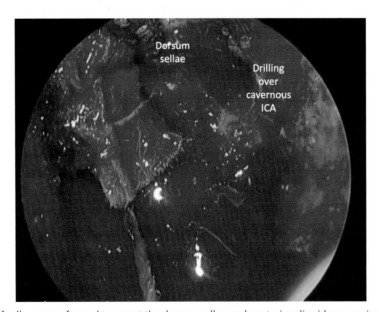

Figure 17-3b. The drilling of sella was performed to resect the dorsum sellae and posterior clinoid process in extradural fashion. It allows to access the interpeduncular cisternal area. The drilling out of bone over the siphon of ICA and paraclival ICA is not mandatory. The midline of dorsum could be drilled out with the elevation of sellar dura after drilling the sella and upper clivus. Venous bleeding from basilar plexus could not be avoided due to the adhesion of skull base bone and periosteal layer of dura.

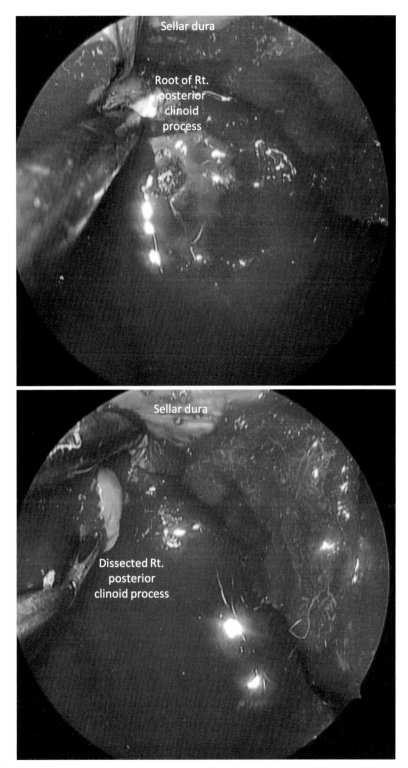

Figure 17-3c. And then, the bony structures covering the cavernous sinus were completely drilled out. The posterior clinoid could be mobilized from the dura and removed with extradural fashion.

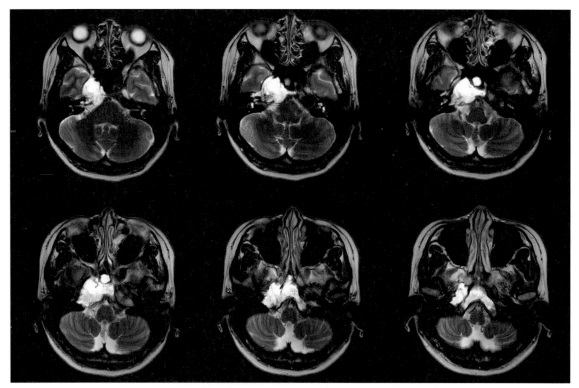

Figure 17-3d-1. A case of chordoma invading cavernous sinus, clivus and medial petrous bone upto internal auditory canal.

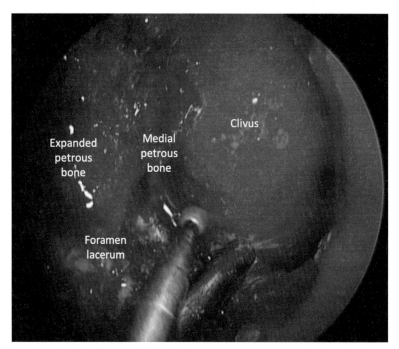

Figure 17-3d-2. The tumor invaded medial petrous area accessible by the drilling of expanded medial petrous bone between clivus and paraclival ICA under the view of 30 degree endoscope.

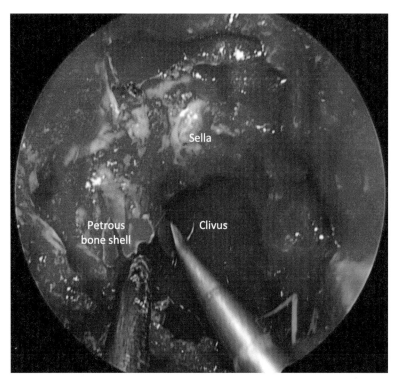

Figure 17-3d-3. The bone shell was dissected to expose the dura covering the tumor.

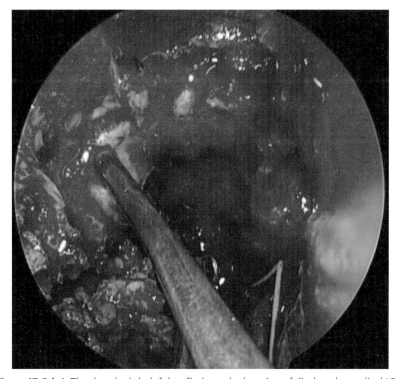

Figure 17-3d-4. The doppler is helpful to find out the location of displaced paraclival ICA.

4. Intradural dissection

Almost targeted tumors for trans-clival and petrous approach are the tumors originating from the skull base bone or intracranial extra-axial tumors. Therefore, the extra-dura or -arachnoid dissection is the key to preserve or improve the neurological status.

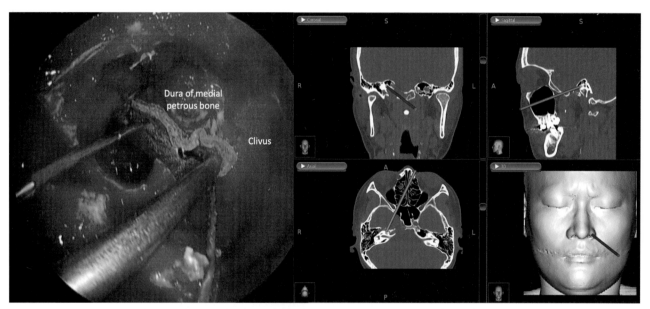

Figure 17-4a. A case of chordoma presented in figure 17-3d-1. The meningeal layer of dura over the medial petrous bone was intact and no cerebrospinal fluid leakage occurred after gross total resection. The indicator of the intraoperative navigation system showed the lateral border of the tumor, just in front of internal auditory canal.

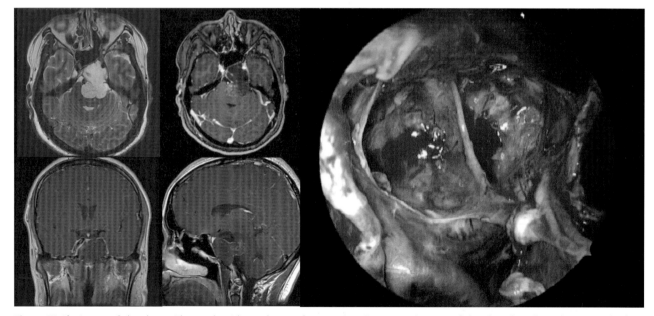

Figure 17-4b. A case of chordoma. The arachnoid membrane of prepontine cistern was intact and the played a role as the protective barrier for the brainstem and major vessels.

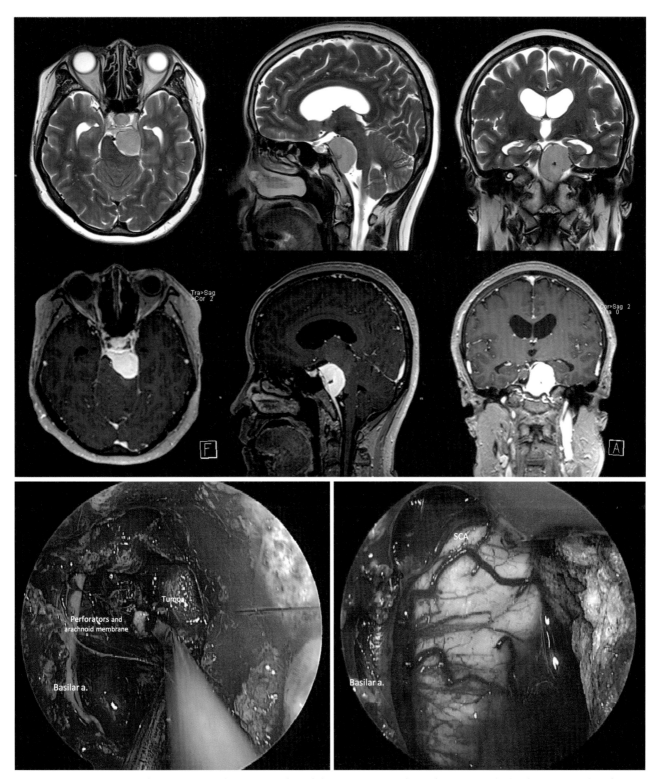

Figure 17-4c. A case of clival meningioma. The extra-arachnoid dissection was performed to protect the basilar artery and perforators and clear brainstem surface was preserved.

III. Tips and summary

The ventral medial petrous area is the very small bony area and the underlying dura composing the basilar plexus bringing profuse bleeding. It is not easy to remove the intracranial tumor beyond the Dorello's canal or attached to the posterior dura of the para-clival ICA without the destruction of petrous bone and displacement of them by the tumor, because the transposition of paraclival ICA is limited by the lateral petrous bone and the thick fibrous tissue of the fora-men lacerum and it is difficult to control the bleeding from the meningohypophyseal artery originated from the dorsal side of ICA. The medial trans-petrous ap-proach is not the totally different surgical approach with the transclival approach but its lateral extension following the tumor extent. The most suitable indi-cations for endoscopic transclival and transpetrosal approach are the chordoma, chondrosarcoma, choles-teatoma and clival meningioma.

REFERENCES

1. Shkarubo AN, Koval KV, Shkarubo MA, Chernov IV, Andreev DN, Panteleyev AA. Endoscopic endonasal transclival approach to tumors of the clivus and anterior region of the posterior cranial Fossa: An anatomic study. World Neurosurg 2018;119:e825-41.

2. Jecko V, Sesay M, Liguoro D. Anatomical location of the abducens nerves (VI) in the ventral approach of clival tumors. Surg Radiol Anat 2020;42(11):1371-5.

Video 17-1. An operation clip of the transclival approach

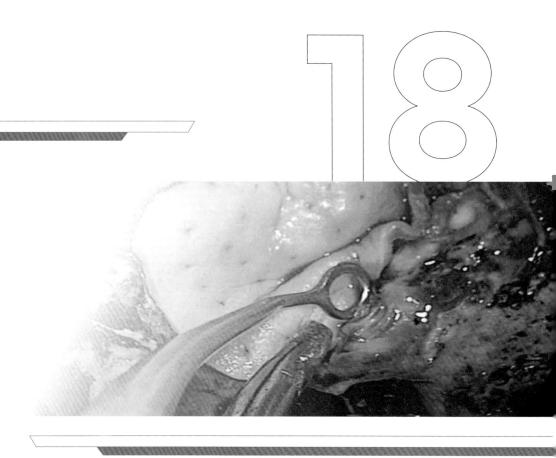

18

ENDOSCOPIC TRANS-TUBERCULAR APPROACH

Young-Hoon Kim M.D., Ph.D.

I. Introduction

The endoscopic skull base approach has shown the advantages to avoid craniotomy, to minimize brain retraction, and to access from the origin of the tumor compared to the conventional skull base approach. Especially, approaching the tumor from below has some benefits such as the possibility of early removal of the bone adjacent to the origin dura, early devascularization of the tumor, and better visualization and preservation of the superior hypophyseal arteries supplying optic chiasma.

The endoscopic trans-tubercular approach is the most basic extended approach beyond the trans-sellar approach, and can be accessed by removing only the tuberculum, planum sphenoidale, and infero-medial part of the optic canal. This approach allows the easier removal of tumors invading the optic canal and the better accessing the hypothalamus and tumor adhesion sites from the bottom. The optimal indication of the endoscopic trans-tubercular approach is the tumor located above the diaphragm or in the third ventricle, i.e. tuberculum sellae meningioma or craniopharyngioma (**Figure 18-1**).

However, it is difficult to completely remove the tumor that grew beyond the lateral of the optic nerve or the intracerebral arteries with the endoscopic approach alone. The other disadvantages of this approach include postoperative CSF leakage, limited surgical freedom, and the inability to gain adequate

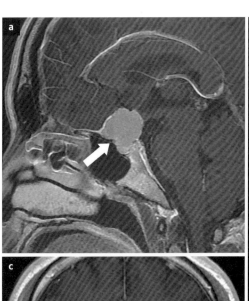
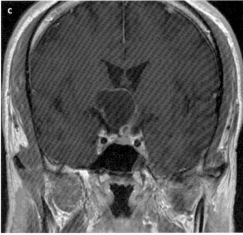
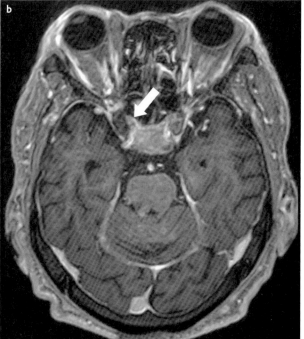

Figure 18-1. (a) The sagittal T1-weighted gadolinium enhanced MRI shows the 3 cm-sized tuberculum sellae meningioma. The white arrow depicts the direction of the endoscopic trans-tubercular approach. (b) The white arrow shows the tumor invading the right optic canal in the axial T1-weighted gadolinium enhanced MRI. (c) The another coronal T1-weighted gadolinium enhanced MRI presents the 3.5 cm-sized craniopharyngioma originated from the pituitary stalk, which is located in the third ventricle.

vascular control in case of major vascular injury.

II. Procedures

1. Nasoseptal flap harvest and intranasal procedures

The first step of the extended endoscopic approach is harvesting of the vascular pedicled nasoseptal flap. The size of the flap is better as it is wider to completely cover the defects of the skull base and not to make dead space between the flap and sphenoid sinus (**Figure 18-2**).

The sphenoidectomy should be sufficiently wide to fully expose both cavernous sinuses and optic canals, tuberculum, and planum sphenoidale. Especially, it is necessary to make sure of the upper and more lateral exposure compared to the traditional trans-sphenoidal approach. If necessary, the posterior ethmoidec-

tomy is recommended.

2. Bony and dural opening

The boundary of the bony opening include the sellar floor, tuberculum sellae, planum sphenoidale, medial opticocarotid recess, and proximal walls of the optic canals (**Figure 18-3a**). The most important bony landmarks are the medial opticocarotid recess and the lateral limbus sphenoidale. Sufficient removal of these two parts can clearly identify the tumors that invade the optic canals.

Dural opening starts at the midline of the suprasellar space and proceeds upward across the superior intercavernous sinus. When cutting the sinus, sufficient coagulation should be performed using a suitable endoscopic bipolar cautery device. Then, the dural incision is extended laterally so that the tumor and optic nerves are sufficiently exposed (**Figure 18-3b**).

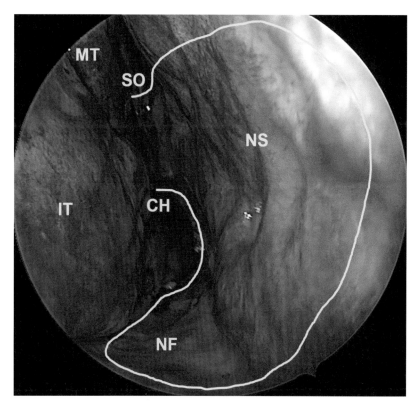

Figure 18-2. The yellow line depict the margin of the nasoseptal flap.
CH, choana; IT, inferior turbinate; MT, middle turbinate; NF, nasal floor; NS, nasal septum; SO, sphenoid sinus ostium

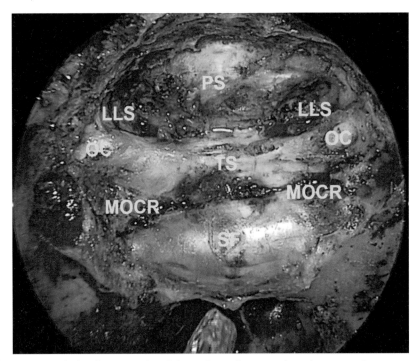

Figure 18-3a. This endoscopic view depicts bony opening of the endoscopic trans-tubercular approach.
LLS, lateral limbus sphenoidale; MOCR, medial opticocarotid recess; OC, optic canal; PS, planum sphenoidale; SF, sellar floor; TS, tuberculum sellae

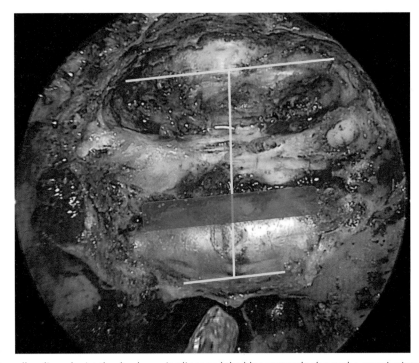

Figure 18-3b. The yellow lines depict the dural opening lines and the blue rectangle shows the superior intercavernous sinus.

3. Intradural procedures (for the tuberculum sellae meningioma)

After opening the dura, the dural tack-up sutures are recommended to maximize the lateral view of the tumors and to prevent epidural bleeding (**Figure 18-4a**). After exposure of the tumor, the biopsy and debulking can be achieved by a suction, microscissors, or ultrasonic aspirators. The subarachnoid dissection and microsurgical principles are always respected and the arachnoid membrane of the tumor is used to protect critical structures such as the superior hypophyseal arteries, the pituitary stalk and gland, the optic nerves, and chiasm. When the tumor is large, the adhesion between the tumor and the anterior cerebral arteries and their branches should be considered. If the tumor involves the optic canal, the optic sheath is opened with angled scissors under angled endoscopic visualization. In most cases, you should observe the medial and inferior side of the optic canal (**Figure 18-4b**).

4. Intradural procedures (for the craniopharyngioma)

In case of the craniopharyngioma, after dural opening, the relationship between the tumor and surrounding neurovascular structures including optic chiasm and nerves, superior hypophyseal arteries, diaphragm sellae, pituitary gland and stalk, and other intracerebral arteries. The basic principles of resection are identical to those of conventional microsurgical removal; that is the extracapsular sharp dissection without injuring neurovascular structures (**Figure 5A**). Most of the craniopharyngiomas tend to show severe adhesion to the hypothalamus (**Figure 5B**). During or after removal of the tumor, the pia mater protecting perforating arteries from the large intracerebral arteries should be protected (**Figure 18-5c**).

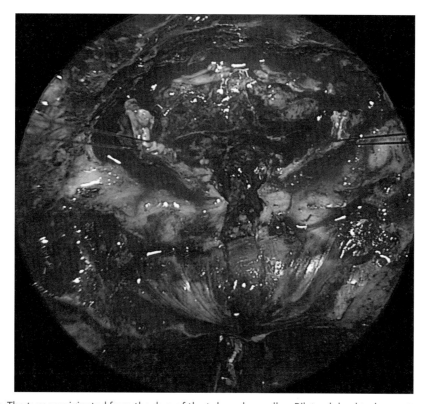

Figure 18-4a. The tumor originated from the dura of the tuberculum sellae. Bilateral dural tack-up sutures were done.

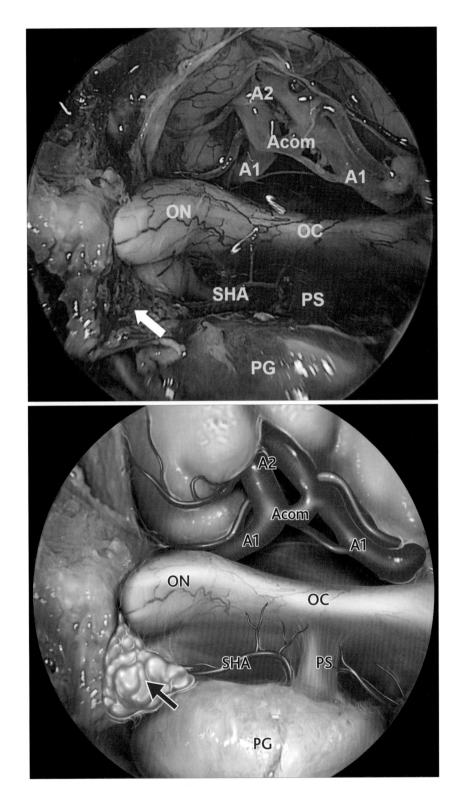

Figure 18-4b. The residual tumor was observed in the medial and inferior side of the optic canal.
A1, anterior cerebral artery; Acom, anterior communicating artery; OC, optic chiasm; ON, optic nerve; PG, pituitary gland; PS, pituitary stalk; SHA, superior hypophyseal artery

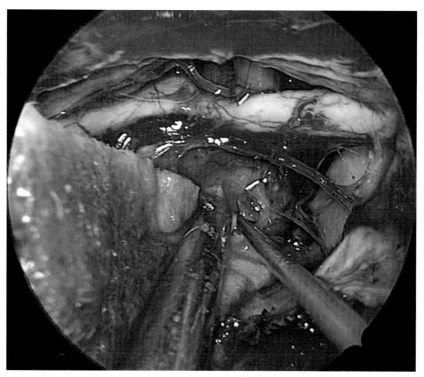

Figure 18-5a. The extracapsular sharp dissection should be performed for not injuring the superior hypophyseal arteries.

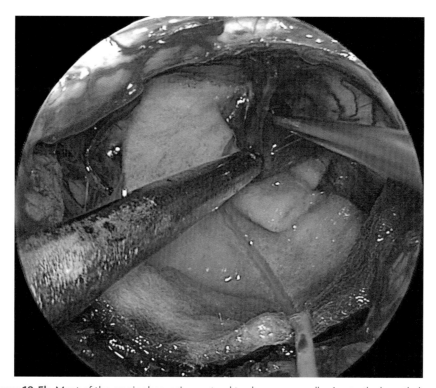

Figure 18-5b. Most of the craniopharyngiomas tend to show severe adhesion to the hypothalamus

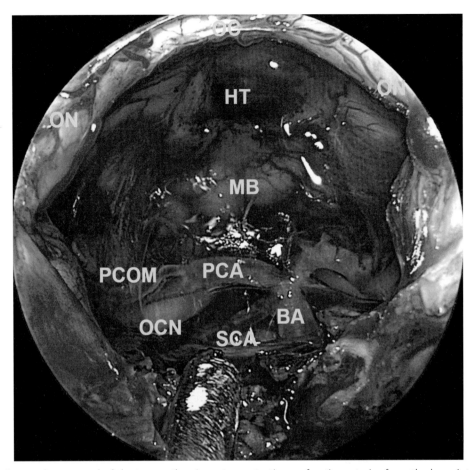

Figure 18-5c. During or after removal of the tumor, the pia mater protecting perforating arteries from the large intracerebral arteries should be protected.

BA; basilar artery, HT; hypothalamus, MB; mammillary body, OC; optic chiasm, OCN; oculomotor nerve, ON; optic nerve, PCA; posterior cerebral artery, PCOM; posterior communicating artery, SCA; superior cerebellar artery

5. Closure and skull base reconstruction

The outcome of the extended endoscopic approach depends on how complete surgeons prevent the CSF leakage. The basic principle of the skull base reconstruction followed by the endoscopic approach is the multi-layer technique.

The surgical cavity or dead space can be filled with the autologous abdominal fat graft or the absorbable gelatin powder (Gelfoam®). The dural layer is reconstructed by the autologous fascia lata graft, dural regeneration matrices (Duragen®), or acellular dermal matrices (Megaderm®) (**Figure 18-6a**). After sealing with fibrin sealant patch (Tachosil®), the injectable hydroxyapatite cement (Hydroset®) can be applied for bony reconstruction (**Figure 18-6b**). Finally, you can cover the surgical site with a previously harvested nasoseptal flap (**Figure 18-6c**).

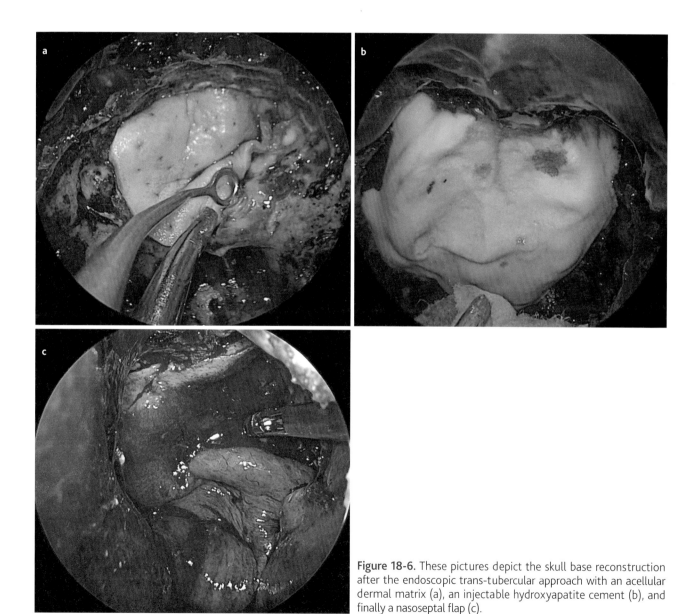

Figure 18-6. These pictures depict the skull base reconstruction after the endoscopic trans-tubercular approach with an acellular dermal matrix (a), an injectable hydroxyapatite cement (b), and finally a nasoseptal flap (c).

223

III. Tips and summary

1. The endoscopic trans-tubercular approach is one of the most basic and widely used extended endoscopic skull base approaches and the optimal indications of this approach include the tuberculum sellae meningioma and craniopharyngioma.
2. Wide vascularized nasoseptal flap and sphenoidotomy are essential.
3. The medial opticocarotid recess and lateral limbus sphenoidale are the most important bony landmarks.
4. The medial and inferior side of the optic canal should be explored for complete removal of the tuberculum sellae meningioma.
5. The multi-layer techniques including dural, bony and mucosal layer reconstructions are needed for the skull base reconstruction after the endoscopic trans-tubercular approach.

REFERENCES

1. Ditzel Filho LFS, Prevedello DM, Jamshidi AO, Dolci RL, Kerr EE, Campbell R, et al. Endoscopic endonasal approach for removal of tuberculum sellae meningiomas. Neurosurg Clin N Am 2015;26(3):349-61.

2. Kong D-S, Hong C-K, Hong SD, Nam D-H, Lee J-I, Seol HJ, et al. Selection of endoscopic or transcranial surgery for tuberculum sellae meningiomas according to specific anatomical features: a retrospective multicenter analysis (KOSEN-002). J Neurosurg 2018;130(3):838-47.

3. Kassam AB, Gardner PA, Snyderman CH, Carrau RL, Mintz AH, Prevedello DM. Expanded endonasal approach, a fully endoscopic transnasal approach for the resection of midline suprasellar craniopharyngiomas: a new classification based on the infundibulum. J Neurosurg 2008;108(4):715-28.

4. Dho Y-S, Kim YH, Se Y-B, Han DH, Kim JH, Park C-K, et al. Endoscopic endonasal approach for craniopharyngioma: the importance of the relationship between pituitary stalk and tumor. J Neurosurg 2018;129(3):611-9.

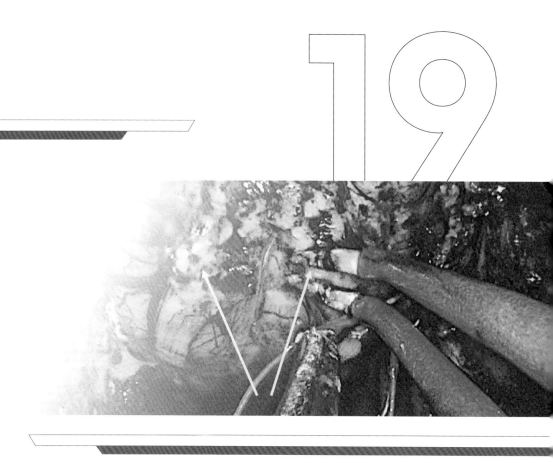

ENDOSCOPIC ENDONASAL TRANSCRIBRIFORM APPROACH

Sang Duk Hong M.D., Ph.D.

I. Introduction

The lesions of the anterior skull base have been traditionally approached through anterior craniotomy or combined craniofacial resections (CFR). Transfacial approaches are cosmetically undesirable. And transcranial approaches often require significant brain retraction and obliteration of the anterior portion of the sagittal sinus. The morbidities such as frontal lobe edema, hematoma, cerebrospinal fluid (CSF) leak, infection, pneumocephalus and skin necrosis can happen in up to 35% of cases. Furthermore, en bloc resection that is thought to be the main benefit of CFR is not always possible because of limited visualization of orbital apex, frontal recess and sphenoid sinus.

With advances in endoscopic skull base surgery, minimally invasive endoscopic approaches to the anterior cranial fossa have been described. The transcribriform approach is the endonasal endoscopic approach through the cribriform plate and fovea ethmoidalis that avoids any facial incision, brain retraction and damage to sagittal sinus with good visualization. Extent of endoscopic transcribriform approach could be from the posterior wall of the frontal sinus back to the planum sphenoidale and between the orbits (**Figure 19-1**).

The Main indication of transcribriform approach is the sinonasal malignancy invading anterior skull base (**Figure 19-2a**) such as squamous cell carcinoma, olfactory neuroblastoma, adenocarcinoma, malignant melanoma, etc. Other pathologies including meningoencephalocele (**Figure 19-2b**), schwannoma and olfactory groove meningioma (**Figure 19-2c**) could be treated by this approach.

This chapter shows the surgical technique especially for sinonasal malignancy invading anterior skull base that is the most common indication of transcribriform approach.

1. Preoperative workup

The otorhinolaryngologic evaluation with cranial nerve examination should be performed. Nasopharyngoscopy must be performed and surgeons should identify whether a tumor invades the contralateral nasal septum or not in order to decide availability of pedicled nasoseptal flap (NSF).

Imaging studies include computed tomography (CT) and magnetic resonance imaging (MRI) of paranasal

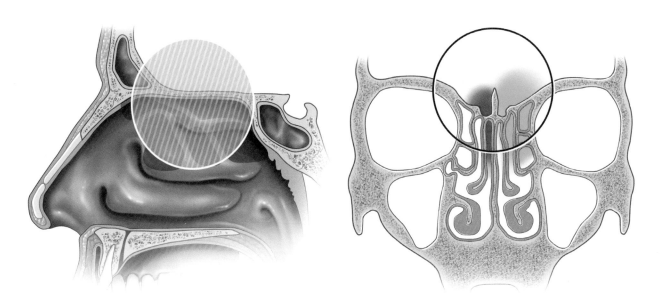

Figure 19-1. Surgical Extents of transcribriform approach.

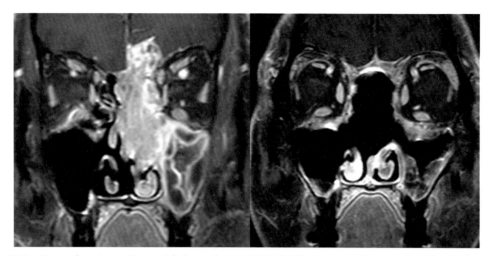

Figure 19-2a. Pre- and postoperative gadolinium enhanced MRI of Olfactory neuroblastoma invading the frontal lobe

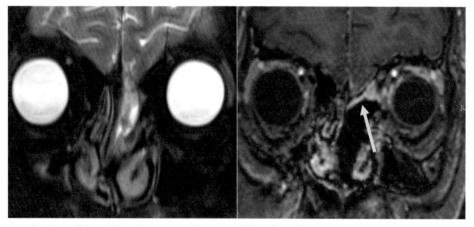

Figure 19-2b. Preoperative T2 weighted MRI showed meningoencephalocele and postoperative gadolinium enhanced T1 weighted MRI showed complete resection of mass and well reconstructed skull base. Arrow indicates nasoseptal flap.

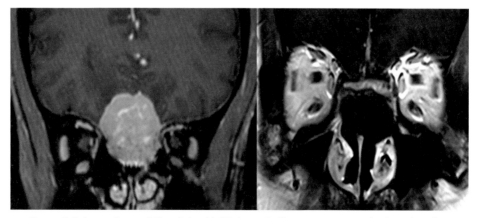

Figure 19-2c. Preoperative gadolinium enhanced T1 weighted MRI showed olfactory groove meningioma invading sinonasal cavity. Postoperative MRI showed complete resection with a well reconstructed skull base.

sinuses, orbits and the brain. If available, preoperative biopsy in the office is needed. If lesion is revealed to be a malignant tumor after biopsy, positron emission tomography (PET)/CT scan should be considered to evaluate regional and distant metastasis.

II. Procedure

1. General anesthesia and preparation

After induction of general anesthesia, intravenous antibiotics that cross the blood-brain barrier are used. Lumbar drain is not routinely used. The nasal mucosa is decongested with 1:5000~1:10000 epinephrine soaked Cottonoids. The patient is positioned with the head turned slightly to the right and extended about 30 degrees to facilitate exposure of the subfrontal anterior cranial fossa. The head is elevated above the heart to help with venous drainage. Head fixation is usually not used. The lateral thigh and abdomen are prepped for autologous fascia lata or fat grafts. After preparation and draping, the navigation system is calibrated and tested. Intraoperative neuromonitoring could be used in severe brain invading tumors or large olfactory groove meningioma. Using a 0 degree 4-mm rigid endoscope, the mucosa adjacent to sphenopalatine and ethmoidal arteries is injected with a 1:100000 epinephrine.

2. Making proper flap

The first step to be performed is to prepare the proper flap for the skull base reconstruction. Therefore, the procedure starts with the creation of a pedicled NSF which is used at the end of the surgery to reconstruct the anterior skull base. If unilateral resection is planned for early staged malignancy, ipsilateral NSF could be elevated. However, contralateral NSF is usually prepared because of oncologic safety.

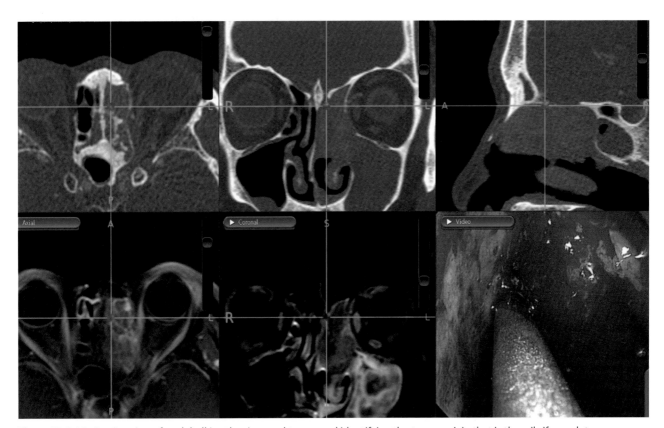

Figure 19-3. Navigation view after debulking the sinonasal tumor and identifying the tumor origin that is the cribriform plate.

When making NSF, it is better to include nasal floor for wider flap and extend to caudal end for longer flap. NSF can be stored in the maxillary sinus or in the nasopharynx during tumor removal. If extensive tumor involvement to the nasal septum, lateral nasal wall flap or pericranial flap could be used.

3. Tumor origin identification and Tumor debulking

Tumor resection starts with endoscopic transnasal debulking of the tumor with a 4-mm microdebrider or Coblator to allow a progressive centrifugal exposure of the margins or stalk of tumors (**Figure 19-3**).

4. Complete spheno-ethmoidectomy with Draf III

The anterior and posterior ethmoidectomy and removal of the middle and superior turbinate are needed to skeletonize the entire anterior skull base until the anterior aspect of the planum sphenoidale is reached. The first olfactory filament is identified at the top of the olfactory cleft, which delineates the posterior limit of the frontal sinus drilling. Draf IIB for unilateral CFR or Draft III for bilateral CFR is performed depending on tumor extension. Draf III starts by localizing the fron-

tal recess bilaterally (in-to-out technique). Superior and anterior septectomy is performed anterior to the cribriform plate that is anterior resection margin of tumor. High speed drill is then used to make and enlarge the common frontal sinusotomy after removing the intersinus septation. Posterior wall of common frontal sinus is visualized (**Figure 19-4**).

5. Endoscopic transnasal craniectomy

A drill and suction are placed through each nostril and endoscopic transnasal craniectomy started bilaterally. The drilling begins at the posterior portion of frontal recess and continues posteriorly to the planum sphenoidale. The lateral limit of the bone removal is the border between the cribriform plate and lamina papyracea. In this point, undermining between dura and skull base bones in lateral fovea ethmoidalis is important to tuck the fascia lata afterwards when reconstruction reconstre (**Figure 19-5**). The crista galli is then drilled out in the midline. Residual thin pieces of bone can be removed with curette or Kerrison rongeurs. The anterior and posterior ethmoidal arteries are identified and cauterized with bipolar diathermy (**Figure 19-6**).

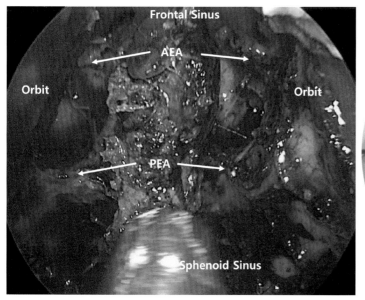
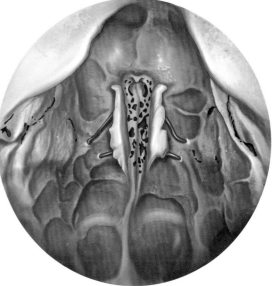

Figure 19-4. 0 degree endoscopic view after bilateral sphenoethmoidectomy with Draf III.

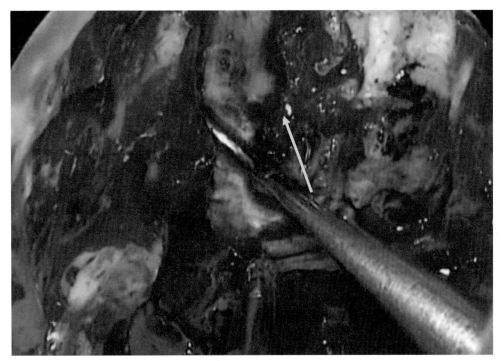

Figure 19-5. Exposing the right anterior ethmoidal artery (AEA) and periorbita. After that, we can safely cauterize and divide the AEA.

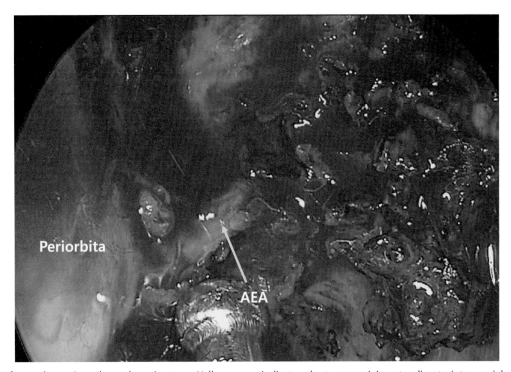

Figure 19-6. After endoscopic endonasal craniectomy. Yellow arrow indicates the tumor origin extending to intracranial space. The instrument undermined space between dura and skull base bone for tucking the fascia lata when doing multilayer reconstruction.

6. Resection of dura with intradural tumor

The lateral dural margin is initially resected just medial to the junction of the lamina papyracea or medial orbital wall periosteum and the fovea ethmoidalis. En bloc resection of the entire specimen is performed in an anterior to posterior direction with the specimen gradually dropping inferiorly into the nose. The excised specimen includes the dura, bilateral cribriform plates with olfactory bulbs, and intracranial tumors. Even if the dura appears uninvolved, it is better to be opened for examination of the olfactory nerves and dura to ensure the absence of intracranial disease. Bipolar cautery is used to control any intracranial bleeding. Adjacent brain parenchyme are meticulously inspected and frozen biopsy from dural margin, olfactory bulb endings and septum are obtained (**Figure 19- 7a, 7b**).

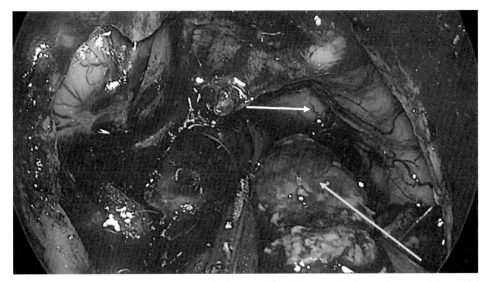

Figure 19-7a. En bloc resection of dura and intracranial tumor (yellow arrow). White arrow indicates the normal frontal lobe parenchyme.

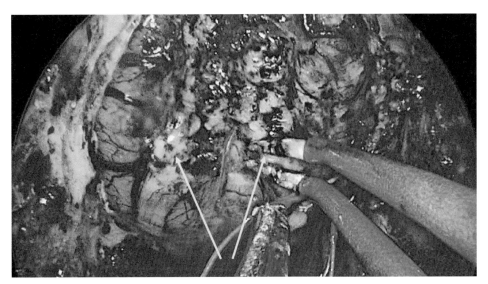

Figure 19-7b. Endoscopic view after en bloc tumor resection and performing meticulous bleeding control by bipolar cauterization. Yellow arrows indicate olfactory bulb margins that confirm negative tumor cells by frozen biopsy.

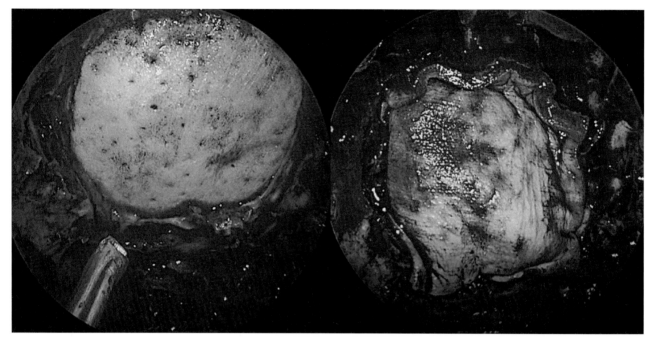

Figure 19-8a. Multilayer reconstruction with acellular dermal graft (Megaderm). Underlay graft (left side) and overlay graft (right side) were done. It is important to tuck the graft between dura and bone.

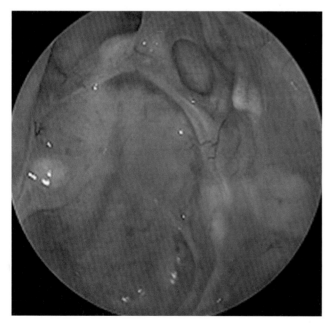

Figure 19-8b. Postoperative endoscopic view showed well healed nasoseptal flap and patent frontal sinus.

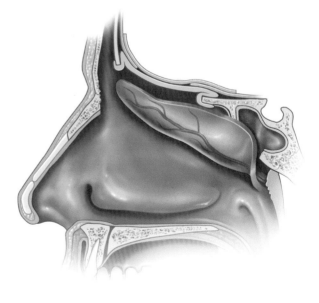

Figure 19-8c. Multilayer reconstruction with Pedicled naso-septal flap

7. Reconstruction

The defect after transcribriform approach may be quite large and the dead space under the brain could be large especially in extensive intracranial involving tumors or olfactory groove meningioma.

Diverse techniques and graft materials can be used for reconstruction. Autologous and homologous fascia lata, acellular dermal allografts, septal cartilage or bone, dural substitutes and other numerous synthetic materials have been used.

Most popular technique is the inlay and overlay autologous fascia lata or acellular dermal grafting and covering pedicled NSF over them (**Figure 19-8**). Although some authors recommend gasket-seal closure using septal bone or Medpor for large cribriform defect, I don't use the free bone graft for patients treated for malignant tumor because of possible osteoradionecrosis after postoperative radiation therapy. After covering NSF on the overlay graft, fibrin sealant such as DuraSeal could be used. However, I preferred solid packing with Merocel to prevent possible downward herniation of the frontal lobe and detaching the flap on the skull base.

III. Tip & Summary

1. Skilled endoscopic skull base teams can safely treat most anterior skull base tumors while maintaining oncologic principles by using endoscopic transcribriform approach.
2. In malignant sinonasal tumor invading skull base, purely endoscopic transcribriform approach allows faster recovery, decreased hospital stay, decreased complication rates and comparable oncologic outcomes with external CFR.
3. Transcribriform approach is the best indication for sinonasal extending olfactory groove meningioma. However, it is not the standard of care for olfactory groove meningioma because of relatively higher cerebrospinal fluid leakage (up to 20%).
4. Early staged olfactory neuroblastoma could be treated by unilateral transcribriform approach to preserve olfaction.
5. Transcribriform approach is not appropriate for dermal involvement, extensive intracranial extension, extraocular muscle invasion and extensive frontal or infratemporal fossa involvement.

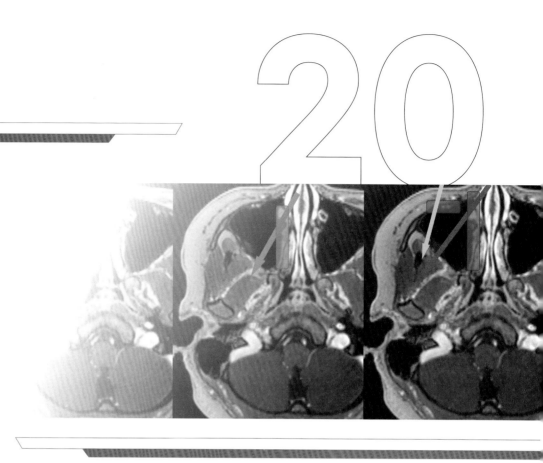

20

TRANSPTERYGOID APPROACH AND CAVERNOUS SINUS

Ju Hyung Moon M.D.

I. Introduction

Endoscopic endonasal transpterygoid approaches imply a corridor that transgresses the pterygoid process. The paired pterygoid processes comprise medial and lateral plates that descend perpendicular from the body of sphenoid bone. The plates are fused at their anterior cephalic aspect, the pterygoid process base. From a ventral perspective, this area contains three important foramina located from superolateral to inferomedial: foramen rotundum, vidian canal, and palatovaginal canal. Due to important anatomical relationships, infratemporal fossa (lateral), pterygo-palatine fossa (anterior), Eustachian tube and fossa of Rosenmüller (posterior), and middle cranial fossa (superior), a partial or complete removal of the pterygoid process (i.e., transpterygoid approach) is a common step to an endonasal endoscopic access to the infratemporal, middle, and posterior cranial fossae. Endoscopic endonasal transpterygoid approaches were first described to provide access to the lateral recess of sphenoid sinus. The traditional approaches to the sphenoid and its lateral recess (transantral, transpalatal, transfacial, and transcranial approaches) are considered invasive and disfiguring procedures. The development of intranasal endoscopic techniques offered a practical alternative to the traditional methods and direct access to the sphenoid sinus while preserving nearby anatomical structures. Recent advances in surgical techniques and technological resources in the field of endoscopy have enabled the use of endoscopic endonasal transpterygoid approach to access to the foramen lacerum, petrous internal carotid artery (ICA), Meckel's cave, cavernous sinus, lateral nasopharynx (fossa of Rosenmüller) and infratemporal fossa.

II. Indications

The transpterygoid approach is used as a corridor to reach pathologies of the middle cranial fossa and posterior cranial fossa. Fibro-osseous lesions, juvenile nasopharyngeal angiofibroma, meningo-encephalocele, schwannoma, and inverted papilloma are some examples of the diseases that can originated from or extend into the lateral recess of the sphenoid sinus. Pathologies of the paramedian-lateral structures of the middle cranial base such as the sella, parasellar area, and lateral portion of the cavernous sinus (e.g., invasive pituitary macroadenomas) can be accessed by this approach as well. Furthermore, the transpterygoid approach is indicated as a corridor to target different areas such as the medial petrous apex, infrapetrous region, inferior cavernous sinus, petroclival area, and infratemporal fossa. Lesions that expand the petrous apex toward the clivus and the lateral recess of the sphenoid sinus such as cholesterol granulomas, cholesteatomas, and dermoid tumors, and lesions situated along the medial portion of the petroclival junction such as chondrosarcomas, chordomas, and petroclival meningiomas can be included in these indications (**Figure 20-1**). The indications for this approach de-

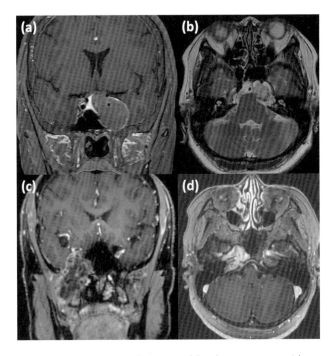

Figure 20-1. Lesions can be assessed by the transpterygoid approach. (a) Pituitary macroadenoma invading right cavernous sinus, (b) Chordoma at left petroclival area, (c) Trigeminal schwannoma involving right middle cranial fossa and inferior temporal fossa, (d) Chondrosarcoma arising from right petroclival junction involving inferior petrous apex.

pend upon the location, type, and consistency of the lesion; they are generally indicated when the neuro-vascular structures are not involved.

III. Procedure

1. Patient Positioning and preparation

- Position: Supine with the head fixed with a Mayfield head holder.
- Body: The body is placed horizontal or in a slight reverse Trendelenburg position (15-30°).
- Head: The head is slightly extended and rotated to the right.
- Abdomen and contralateral thigh are prepped and draped in a sterile fashion in case a fat graft or fascia lata are needed.

2. Nasal Stage

- Before starting the surgical dissection, the surgeon must identify fundamental anatomical landmarks such as the inferior turbinate, the head of the middle turbinate and its attachment to the maxillary bone (axilla of the middle turbinate), the nasal septum, and the uncinate process.
- Middle turbinate is resected (**Figure 20**-2).
- Uncinectomy is carried out. The uncinate process is a C-shaped process of the ethmoid bone, which represents a small part of the medial wall of the maxillary sinus posteriorly to the lacrimal bone and articulates with the axilla of the middle turbinate (**Figure 20**-3).

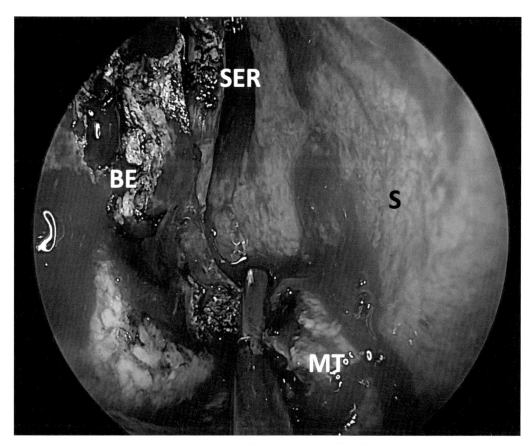

Figure 20-2. Middle turbinectomy (Right)
BE = bulla ethmoidalis; MT = middle turbinate; S = septum; SER= sphenoethmoidal recess.

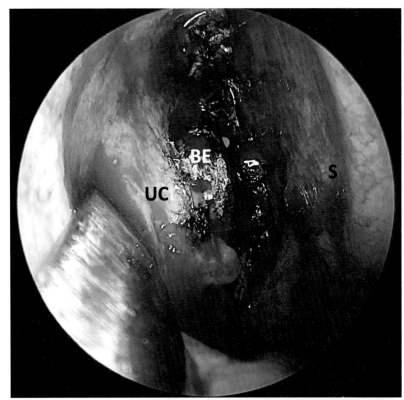

Figure 20-3. Uncinectomy (Right)
BE = bulla ethmoidalis; S = septum; UC = uncinate process.

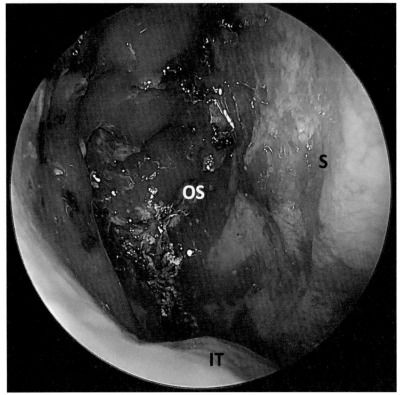

Figure 20-4. Ethmoidectomy (Right)
IT = inferior turbinate; OS = sphenoid ostium; S = septum.

- Maxillary sinus ostium is identified within the concavity designed by the uncinate process.
- Ethmoidectomy is performed: the ethmoidal bulla and supra-bulla cells are both removed. The safe opening of the ethmoidal bulla should be performed starting medially and inferiorly, keeping in mind that the lateral wall of the bulla corresponds to the lamina papyracea of the orbit (**Figure 20-4**).
- A contralateral nasoseptal flap is harvested
- Complete a septectomy by resecting the posterior nasal septum.
- Opening of sphenoid sinus is performed by removing the anterior wall of the sphenoid sinus.

3. Maxillary Sinus Stage

- A wide maxillary antrostomy is carried out.

The antral surgical corridor should be adapted to the intended target area, and its extent can be estimated preoperatively. Endoscopic endonasal transpterygoid approaches to the pterygopalatine fossa, lateral recess of the sphenoid sinus, and petrous apex and Meckel's cave target areas above the level of the vidian canal. Their antral access only requires a maxillary antrostomy. An adequate nasoantral window should expose the superior half of the posterior wall of the maxillary sinus when using a 0-degree endoscope. Conversely, access to the infratemporal fossa, lateral nasopharynx implies exposure of a target that extends below the vidian canal; thus, its antral access requires a medial maxillectomy to expose the entire height of the posterior wall of the antrum. A medial maxillectomy should extend from the nasolacrimal duct to the posterior wall of the antrum (anteroposteriorly) and from the inferior orbital wall to the floor of the nasal cavity (cephalocaudally). In addition, extended approaches to the infratemporal fossa and/or middle cranial base or fossa may require an endoscopic Denker's approach or a Caldwell-Luc approach to extend the medial maxillectomy anteriorly and laterally. It should be noted that this extension could be customized to the needs of the case; therefore, in many cases some of the previously mentioned steps may be obviated (**Figure 20-5, 6**).

- The posterior wall of the maxillary sinus is removed by drilling the vertical and orbital processes of the palatine bone (i.e., anterior wall of the sphenopala-

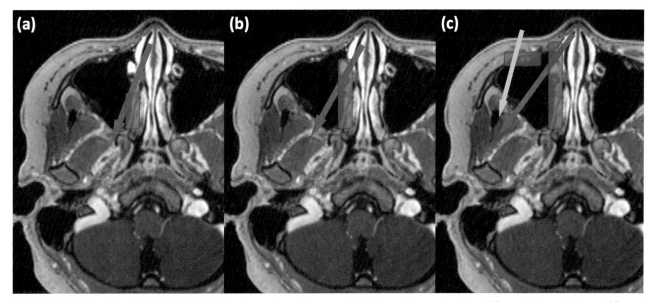

Figure 20-5. Comparison of lateral limits of the transpterygoid approach with maxillary antrostomy (a), medial maxillectomy (b), and Denker's (red arrow) or Caldwell-Luc (yellow arrow) (c) approach. Blue rectangles indicate the bony opening of the maxillary sinus of each approach.

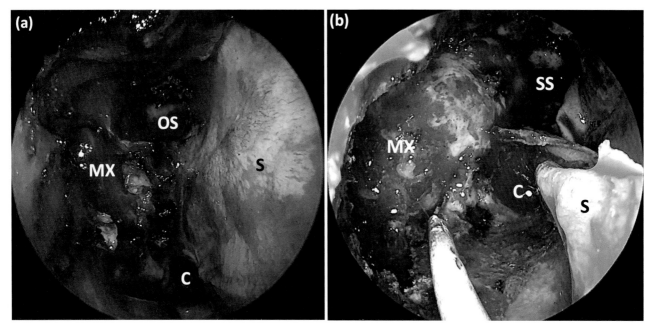

Figure 20-6. Comparison of the endoscopic view after maxillary antrostomy (a) and medial maxillectomy (b) (Right)
C = choana; MX = maxillary sinus; OS = sphenoid ostium; S = septum; SS = sphenoid sinus.

tine foramen).

- The infraorbital neurovascular bundle is identified.
- Sphenopalatine artery is cauterized and divided.
- The periosteal layer covering the pterygopalatine fossa is opened.

4. Exposure of the Pterygopalatine Fossa (PPF) (Figure 20-7)

- The contents of the pterygopalatine fossa are laterally retracted.
- The inferior portion of the medial pterygoid plate is drilled.
- The vidian nerve at the junction of the sphenoid sinus floor and medial pterygoid plate is identified.
- The pterygoid wedge (anterior junction of the medial and lateral pterygoid plates) is identified.
- The foramen rotundum and the maxillary nerve (V2) at the superior margin of the pterygopalatine fossa are identified, by travelling laterally and superiorly toward the inferior orbital fissure.

5. Accessing Cavernous Sinus (Figure 20-8)

- The medial and lateral pterygoid plates are drilled back
- The vidian nerve is exposed back to the junction of the paraclival and lacerum segment of the ICA.
- The quadrangular space is exposed; it is defined by the carotid artery medially and inferiorly, by the maxillary nerve laterally and superiorly by the sixth cranial nerve and the first branch of the trigeminal nerve (V1) (Figure 20-9).

6. Cavernous Sinus Anatomy

The cavernous sinus is a blood-filled dural venous sinus that lies within the middle cranial fossa between the sella medially and the anteromedial temporal lobe laterally. It transmits multiple cranial nerves as well as arteries of the anterior circulation (Figure 20-9). In relation to surgical anatomy, the medial cavernous sinus is that portion of the sinus between the sella in the midline and the ICA laterally. In contrast, the lateral portion of the cavernous sinus is defined as that which

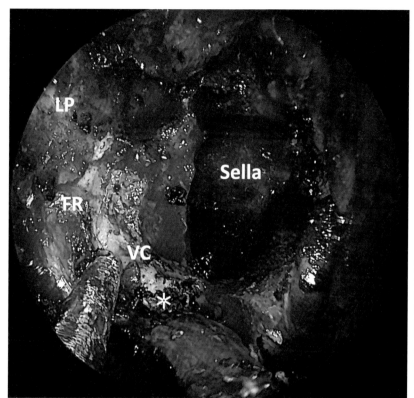

Figure 20-7. Exposure of right pterygopalatine fossa. Sphenopalatine artery is cauterized and cut at the sphenopalatine foramen (asterisk). After inferolateral retraction of the contents of the pterygopalatine fossa, the foramen rotundum & the maxillary nerve (V2) at the superior margin of the fossa and the vidian nerve at the junction of the sphenoid sinus floor is identified.
FR = foramen rotundum; LP = lamina papyracea; VC = vidian canal.

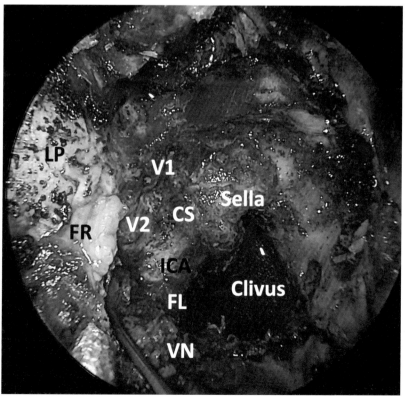

Figure 20-8. Accessing the right cavernous sinus. CS = cavernous sinus; FL = foramen lacerum; FR = foramen rotundum; ICA = internal carotid artery; LP = lamina papyracea; VN = vidian nerve; V1 = ophthalmic nerve; V2 = maxillary nerve.

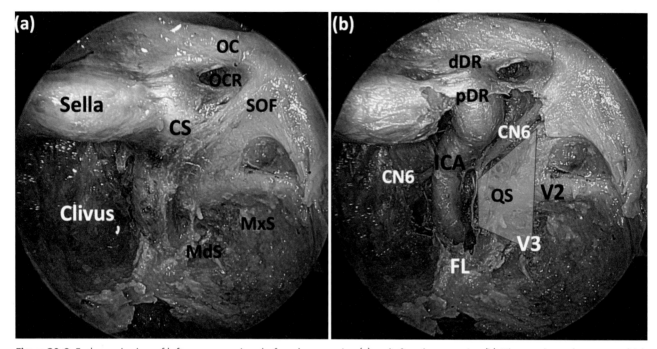

Figure 20-9. Endoscopic view of left cavernous sinus before dura opening (a) and after dura opening (b). The quadrangular space, which is bound by the ICA medially and inferiorly, V2 laterally, and the abducens nerve superiorly, offers direct access to the anteroinferomedial segment of Meckel's cave.

CN = cranial nerve; CS = cavernous sinus; dDR = distal dural ring; FL = foramen lacerum; ICA = internal carotid artery; MxS = maxillary strut; MdS = mandibular strut; OC = optic canal; OCR = lateral opticocarotid recess; pDR = proximal dural ring; QS = quadrangular space; V2 = maxillary nerve; V3 = mandibular nerve.

lies between the ICA, to the boundary of the cavernous sinus laterally at the dura. In the medial portion of the cavernous sinus, there are not any neural structures but several important anatomical structures. The medial wall of the cavernous sinus forms the lateral boundary of the hypophyseal fossa and separates the pituitary gland from the cavernous segment of the ICA and the venous channels. Multiple ligamentous dura-like trabeculae were found connecting and anchoring the cavernous (lateral) surface of the medial wall of the cavernous sinus to the anterior wall, the ICA, the lateral wall, the interclinoid ligament, and the anterior clinoid process, with much variation in shape, size, and trajectory. The inferior hypophyseal artery can be recognized in the medial cavernous sinus (**Figure 20-10**). In the lateral portion of the cavernous sinus, the lateral cavernous sinus is bounded superiorly by the upper cavernous ICA and its distal dural ring,

and inferiorly by the maxillary strut (the bone arising between V1 at the superior orbital fissure and V2 at foramen rotundum) and the V2 segment of the trigeminal nerve. Within these boundaries , there are the ICA and its associated sympathetic plexus, and cranial nerves III (oculomotor nerve), IV (trochlear nerve), V1 (ophthalmic trigeminal nerve), and VI (abducens nerve). Importantly, the abducens nerve runs freely within the cavernous sinus and is medial to cranial nerves III, IV, and V1, which run in the lateral dura leaflet (**Figure 20-11**). The abducens is therefore more prone to injury in EEA to the lateral cavernous sinus, since it is the first cranial nerve encountered within the sinus when approached from an endonasal perspective and its displacement by a mass lesion is not always predictable. The other cranial nerves, however, are on the far (lateral) side of any mass lesion within the cavernous sinus when approached from an endo-

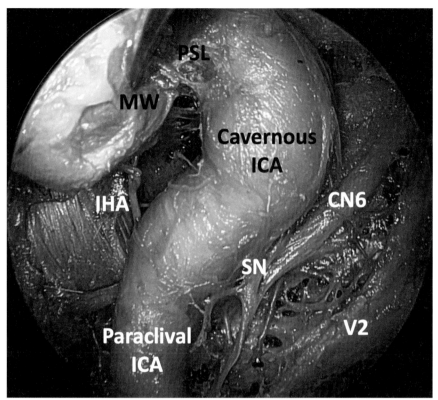

Figure 20-10. Endoscopic view of the medial portion of left cavernous sinus. The medial wall of the cavernous sinus was retracted medially and parasellar ligaments are exposed. Inferior hypophyseal artery is located in the medial portion of cavernous sinus.

CN = cranial nerve; ICA = internal carotid artery; IHA = inferior hypophyseal artery; MW = medial wall of cavernous sinus; PSL = parasellar ligament; SN = sympathetic nerve; V2 = maxillary nerve

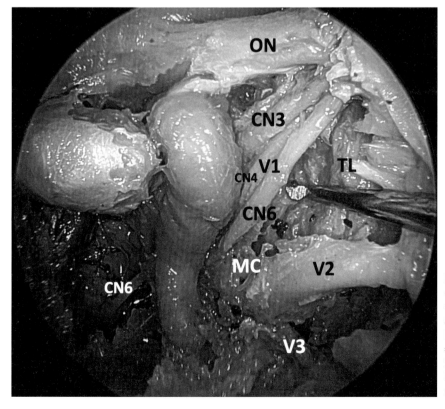

Figure 20-11. Endoscopic view of the lateral portion of left cavernous sinus.

CN = cranial nerve; ICA = internal carotid artery; IHA = inferior hypophyseal artery; MW = medial wall of cavernous sinus; ON = optic nerve; PSL = parasellar ligament; SN = sympathetic nerve; TL = temporal lobe; V1 = optha; mic nerve; V2 = maxillary nerve; V3 = mandibular nerve

nasal endoscopic approach, and this is an advantage over the transcranial route where the cranial nerves are superficial in the field to the pathology and must be worked around.

IV. Pearls

- The entire lateral sphenoid and cavernous sinus can then be visualized and reached surgically with the surgical technique involving a transmaxillary, transpterygoid approach in which the vidian nerve is followed endoscopically back to the lacerum segment of the ICA.
- The posterior wall of the maxillary sinus, vidian foramen, foramen rotundum, Eustachian tube, and sphenoid indentation of ICA are important landmarks.
- The Vidian nerve is a crucial landmark for locating the lacerum segment of the ICA.
- Specialized neuro-endoscopic dissectors, cranial nerve monitoring, neuro-navigation system, and an experienced neurosurgery and otolaryngology team allow safe resection despite multiple intraoperative challenges.
- The angled endoscope and angled instruments facilitate visualization and reach the lateral recess of sphenoid and cavernous sinus.
- The texture and consistency of the tumor dictates the ease and safety of removal. The fibrous nature of cavernous sinus pathologies may preclude a gross-total resection, with the goals of surgery being to decompress the cranial nerves and obtain tissue for pathology, and planned stereotactic or fractionated radiation thereafter, to minimize morbidity.
- The use of flowable hemostatic matrix permits management of venous bleeding including cavernous sinus bleeding.

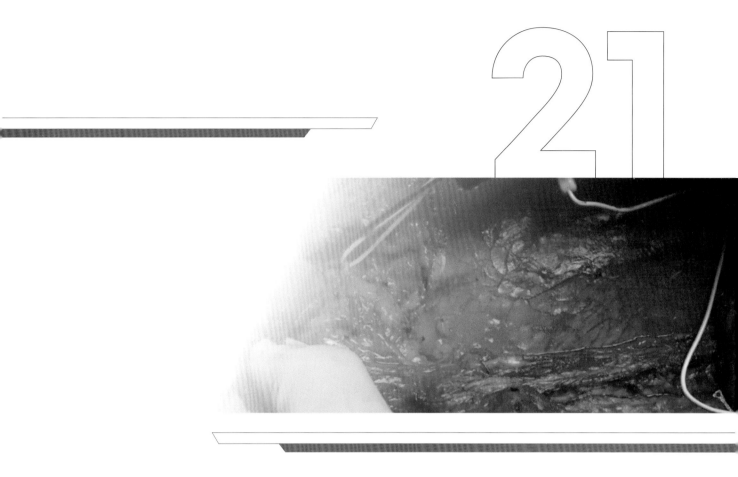

FACIAL NERVE RECONSTRUCTION

Hak Chang M.D., Ph.D.

I. Anatomy of facial nerve

The extratemporal portion of the facial nerve (CN VII) begins at the stylomastoid foramen and extends between the superficial and deep lobes of the parotid gland. Its main branch is divided into two divisions, each of which branches to all parts of the face in five components: the frontotemporal, zygomatic, buccal, marginal mandibular, and cervical (**Figure 21-1**).[1-3]

II. Etiology of facial palsy

The major causes of facial paralysis of adults are in acquired forms, including inflammatory processes, such as Bell's palsy, intracranial lesions, or extracranial trauma (**Table 21-1**). Meanwhile, congenital facial paralysis is the most common form of facial paralysis seen in pediatrics with estimation of 2.0% of live births. The nerves at birth are very superficial and

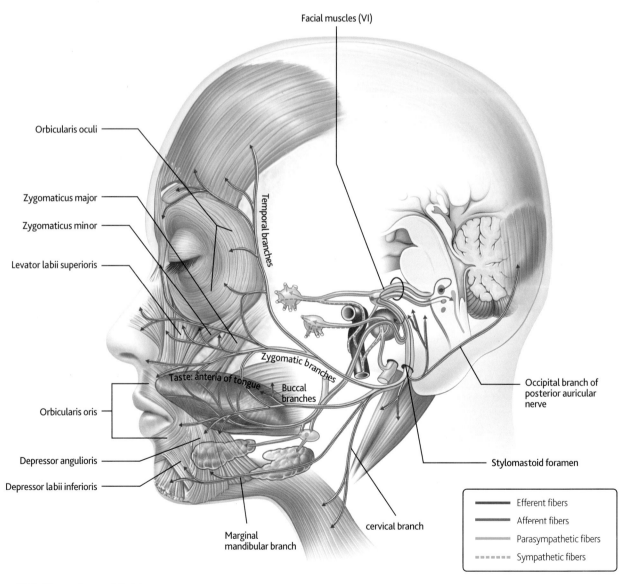

Figure 21-1. The anatomy of facial nerve

Table 21-1. Various causes of facial palsy

Extracranial
Traumatic
Facial lacerations
Blunt forces
Penetrating wounds
Mandible fractures
Iatrogenic injuries
Newborn paralysis
Neoplastic
Parotid tumors
Tumors of the external canal and middle ear
Facial nerve neurinomas
Metastatic lesions
Congenital absence of facial musculature
intratemporal
Traumatic
Fractures of petrous pyrarrid
Penetrating injuries
Iatrogenic injuries
Neoplateic
Glomus tumors
Cholesteatoma
Facial neurinomas
Squamous cell carcinomas
Rhabsomyosarcoma
Arachnoidal cysts
Metastatic
Infectious
Herpes zoster oticus
Acute otitis media
Malignant otitis extema
Idiopathic
Bell palsy
Mekersson-Rosenthal syndrome
Congenital: osteopetrosis
Intracranial
Iatrogenic injury
Neoplastic-benign, malignant, primary, metastatic
Congenital
Absence of motor units
Syndromic
Hemifacial microsomia (unilateral)
Mobius syndrome (bilateral)

can be vulnerable to external compression or surgical intervention. Congenital facial paralysis may be syndromic. The most common syndrome-related unilateral facial paralysis is hemifacial macrosomia, and the most common bilateral paralysis is a result of Möbius syndrome. The functional effects of congenital facial paralysis tend to worsen gradually as the influence of gravity and aging prevails. Throughout all of these areas, facial paralysis constitutes a spectrum of involvement.[4]

III. Treatment options for facial palsy

There are variable approaches to correct facial paralysis, such as medical treatment, surgical decompression, rehabilitation, and reconstructive surgery (Table 21-2). In order to select the most appropriate treatment, multiple factors should be considered, including the patient's chief complaint, age of the patient, duration of the facial paralysis, condition of the facial musculatures, and functionality of the potential donor sites. The optimal goals for surgical treatment include not only the normal appearance at resting state but also the symmetric dynamic movement. The surgical approaches for facial palsy mainly comprises the static and dynamic reconstructions.

For various etiologies and treatment options of facial paralysis, deciding the appropriate treatment approach can be often difficult. The signs and symptoms of facial palsy are highly heterogenous, and the treatment options are extremely diverse. Therefore, we suggest a treatment protocol for facial paralysis with different etiologies (Figure 21-2).

The initial treatment for facial paralysis with idiopathic causes, such as Bell's palsy or Ramsey-Hunt syndrome, includes administration of the steroid or antiviral agents. Electroneurography is suggested within 2 weeks to decide whether decompression is needed in cases with less than 10% of muscle action potential. In iatrogenic facial palsies, immediate exploration is recommended in acute cases with saved facial nerves. If the nerve is confirmed to be sacrificed,

Table 21-2. Treatment options for facial palsy

Steroid/Antivirals
Surgical decompression
Rehabilitation
Reconstructive surgery

Static	Dynamic

Fascial slings to eyelids and mouth
Gold/platinum weight or spring to upper eyelid
Eyelid procedures
  Tarsorrhaphy
  Canthoplasty
  Lower-lid wedge resection
  Lower-lid tendon graft
Cosmetic procedures
  Rhytidectomy
  Rhinoplasty
  Endoscopic browlift
  Blepharoplasty
  Botox
Contralateral myotomy or selective denervation
	Primary repair
	Entubulation enurorrhaphy
	Ipsilateral nerve grafts
	Regional muscle trasfers
	  Temporalis
	  Masseter
	Zygomaticus major muscle plication for partial paralysis
	Nerve transfers (nonemotive voluntary control)
	  Partial hypoglossal
	  Trigeminal motor branch
	  Spinal accessory
	Cross-facial nerve graft (emotive spontaneous control)
	Microneurovascular free tissue transfer
	  Gracilis
	  Latissimus
	  Pectoralis minor
	  Serratus anterior
	  Adductor magnus
	  Rectus femoris
	  Rectus abdominus

reanimation surgeries, such as nerve graft, gold plate insertion, can be considered.

Electromyography is followed up after 2-3 weeks and 3 months later, respectively, to decide whether to continue observation or go on to surgical interventions. The period from the onset of facial palsy to the point where the patient visits the clinic for surgery is important for the selection of operative technique. If the injury has been less than a year when the patient visits the plastic and reconstructive department, nerve transfer or cross-face nerve graft can be considered. However, if the jury has been more than a year, the muscles become irreversibly atrophic and a muscle transfer or static reconstruction can be performed. The effect of the facial musculature can be replaced by static procedures for balance, such as brow lift, gold plate insertion, and lower lid shortening, tendon sling **(Figure 21-3)**.

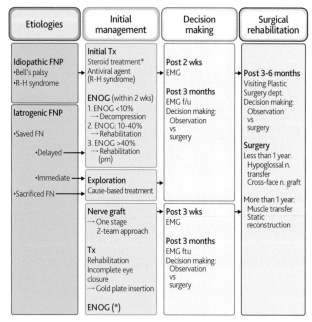

Figure 21-2. Treatment protocol for facial palsy

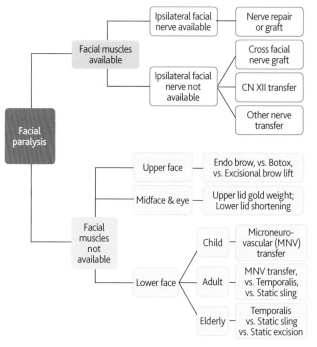

Figure 21-3. Surgical approaches for facial palsy

IV. Surgical techniques

<Static operation>

1. Suprabrow lift

1) Introduction

- Indication

Unilateral frontalis paralysis may cause a difference in brow heights of up to 12 mm. A direct brow lift is best able to correct such large discrepancies.

- Pre-operative preparation or check points

Assessment of the amount of brow depression on the paralyzed side is compared with the normal eyebrow.

2) Procedure

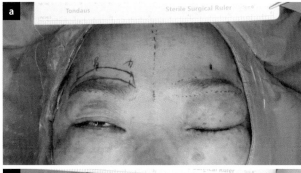
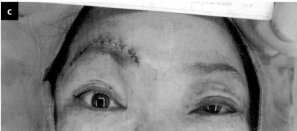
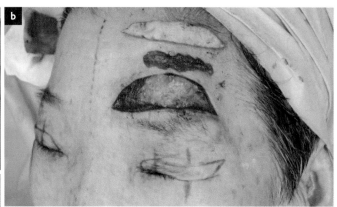

Figure 21-4. (a, b) Direct suprabrow lift involves excision of a segment of skin and frontalis muscle just above and parallel to the eyebrow. The supraorbital nerve should be identified and preserved. (c) A slight overcorrection is required because the excised tissue eventually relaxes in minimal amount over time. Sometimes, periosteo-dermal fixation can be done with non-absorbable sutures to maintain the height more securely.

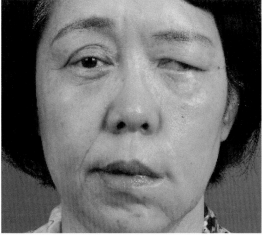
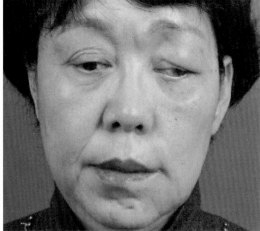

Figure 21-5. Preoperative and postoperative photographs

3) Tip and Summary

This procedure can leave a visible scar above the eyebrow. However, if the incision is placed just along the first line of hair follicles, the resulting scar is usually less noticeable.

2. Subbrow lift

1) Introduction

- Indication

Unilateral laxity in upper eyelid without blepharoptosis can be corrected by subbrow lift.
- Pre-operative preparation or check points

Assessment of the amount of skin laxity on the paralyzed side is compared with the normal eyebrow.

2) Procedure

3. Gold plate insertion

1) Introduction

- Indication

This procedure is directed at overcoming the unopposed action of the levator palpebrae superioris. Because of its relative technical ease and reversibility, lid loading with gold prosthesis is one of the most popu-

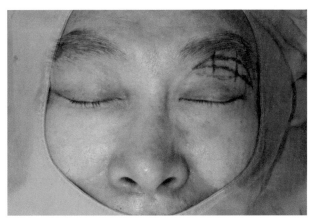

Figure 21-6a. Similar to the suprabrow lift, incision is made just along the lower border of the eyebrow and a segment of skin and soft tissue is excised.

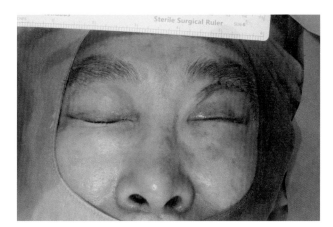

Figure 21-6b. A slight overcorrection is also required.

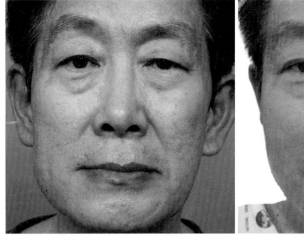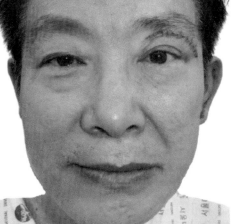

Figure 21-7. Preoperative and postoperative photographs

lar technique.

- Pre-operative preparation or check points

The patient's eyelid configuration is important in determining whether the bulge of the gold weight will be visible when the eye is open. If the amount of exposed eyelid skin above the lashes is more than 5 mm when the eye is open, the gold weight is likely to be noticeable to the patient. If the distance is less than 5mm, the gold weight will roll back and be covered by the supratarsal skinfold.

2) Procedure

After a superior palpebral fold incision is made, the prosthesis is located at the upper half of the tarsal plate and fixated with permanent sutures. Interference with the insertion of Müller muscle should be avoided. After the operation, the patient should be instructed to relax the levator muscle consciously for a few seconds to allow the eyelid to descend (**Figure 21-8**).

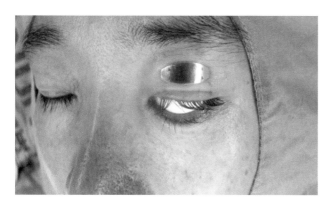

Figure 21-8.

3) Tip and Summary

The lightest weight that will bring the upper eyelid within 2–4 mm of the lower lid and cover the cornea should be used, which is usually around 0.8–1.2 g. As long as the patient has an adequate Bell phenomenon, complete closure is not necessary.[5]

The complications may include excessive capsule formation which causes a visible lump, and irritation of the eye by the weight, and extrusion of the gold plate. In such cases, the weight can easily be repositioned, replaced, or removed (**Figure 21-9**).

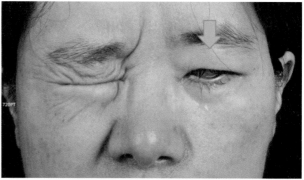
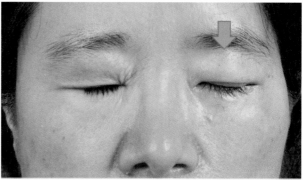

Figure 21-9. Preoperative and postoperative photographs

4. Levator lengthening with conchal cartilage graft

1) Introduction

- Indication

In patients with noticeable bulging at the gold plate insertion site, this alternative method has the advantage of using autogenous material with less noticeable appearance.

2) Procedure

A piece of cartilage is harvested from concha area (**Figure 21-10a, 10b**).

An incision is made at the superior palpebral fold and the levator aponeurosis and Muller's muscles are dissected off from the entire tarsal plate. The harvest conchal cartilage graft is inserted and fixed between the edge of elevated levator aponeurosis and the superior edge of the tarsal plate (**Figure 21-11a, 11b, 11c**).[6]

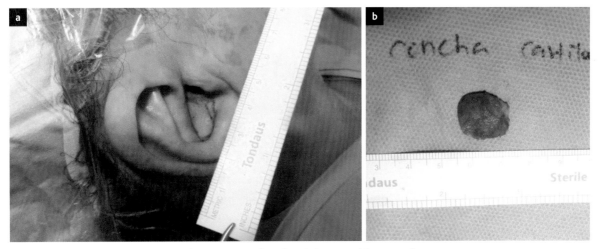

Figure 21-10. A piece of cartilage is harvested from concha area.

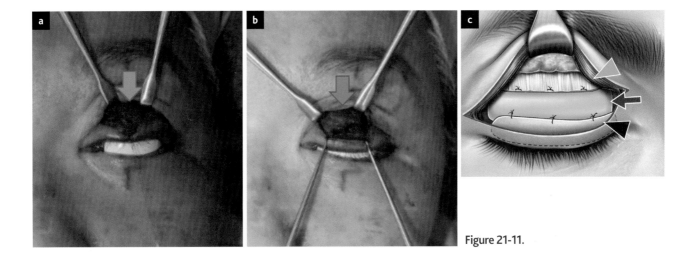

Figure 21-11.

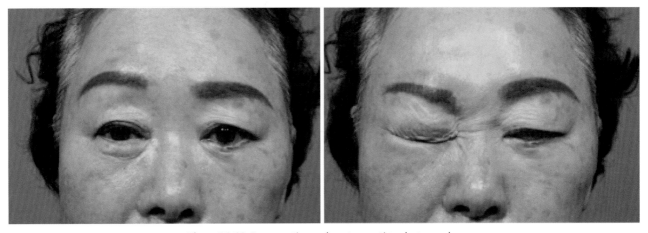

Figure 21-12. Preoperative and postoperative photographs

3) Tip and Summary

The width of conchal cartilage is standardized at minimum of 7 mm to make sure the elongation of the levator aponeurosis.

5. Sling operation

1) Introduction

- Indication

Static slings are used to achieve symmetry at resting state without providing animation. They can be used alone or as an adjunct to dynamic procedures to provide immediate support.

- Pre-operative preparation or check points

The slings can be made of fascia (e.g. tensor fascia latae), tendon (e.g. Palmaris longus), or prosthetic material (e.g. Gore-Tex®).

2) Procedure

A modified Blair incision and an additional naso-labial incision is made and subcutaneous dissection is performed through the incisions up to the oral commissure.

(1) Tenson fascia latae

A tensor fascia latae tendon is harvested from lat-eral thigh and inserted through the dissected area. The distal end of the tendon of the first tendon strip is fixated at the oral commissure and the proximal end is fixated at the deep temporal fascia. The second tendon strip is fixated from the deep soft tissue along the mandible body to the posterior auricular fascia (**Figure 21-13a, 13b**).[7]

(2) Palmaris longus

A Palmaris longus tendon is harvested from the non-dominant forearm in about a 10-15 cm length. Two incisions are made at the wrist level and at the transition zone between the tendon and the muscle belly. Dissection is performed to release the tendon strip from the surrounding soft tissue, and a tendon stripper is used to ligate the proximal end of the tendon (**Figure 21-14a**).

Through the subcutaneous tunnel, the tendon strip is located at an imaginary axis of zygomaticus major from the modiolus to zygomatic arch and extended to the temporal area. The distal end of the tendon strip is fixated at three points around the oral commissure, the upper lip, modiolus, and the lower lip, and the other end is fixated at the deep temporal fascia with non-absorbable sutures (**Figure 21-14b**).

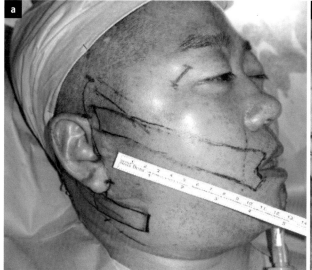
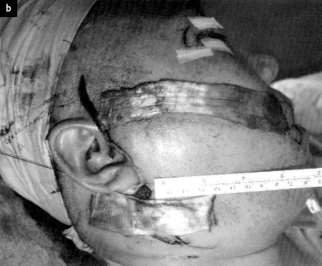

Figure 21-13.

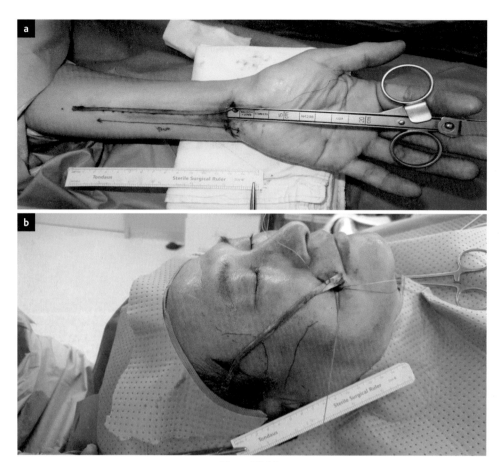

Figure 21-14.

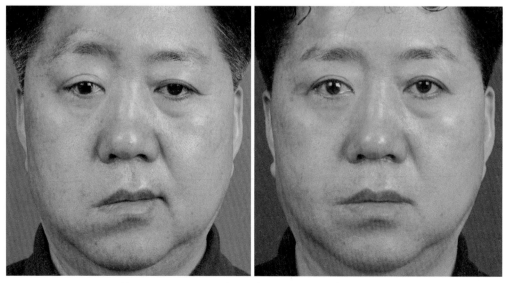

Figure 21-15. Preoperative and postoperative photographs

6. Tip and summary

Multiple grafts can be inserted to provide an even lift to the corner of the mouth and upper lip in a desired direction. The goal is to produce a facial position equal to or slightly overcorrected from the resting position on the normal side. The pulling force should be distributed evenly around the mouth with a little overcorrection. This is done to compensate for the difference in facial tone when the patient is awake and for postoperative stretching. However, special care is needed to avoid inserting the sling too tightly, particularly in the upper lip, which establishes a corridor through which air and liquid can escape.

V. Dynamic operation

1. Cross-face nerve graft and Nerve cross-over

1) Introduction

- Indication

When the ipsilateral proximal facial nerve stump is not usable (brain tumor, head trauma and fractures, Bell's palsy, or surgery) but the facial musculature has not become irreversibly atrophic, a cross-face nerve graft can be very effective. This can preserve the function of the musculature on the paralyzed side and result in a more natural appearance.[8-10]

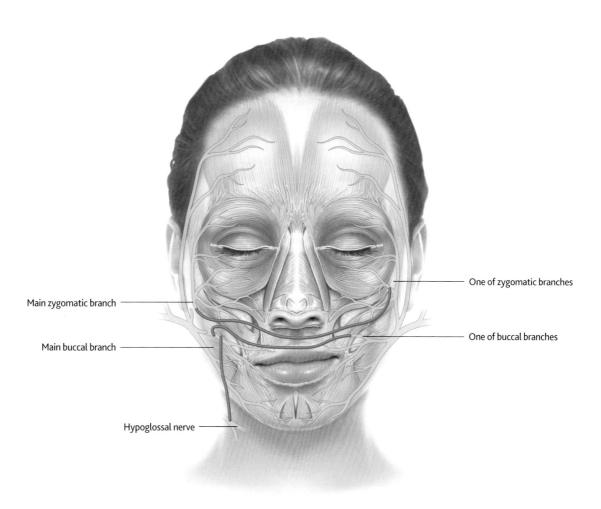

Main zygomatic branch

Main buccal branch

Hypoglossal nerve

One of zygomatic branches

One of buccal branches

Figure 21-16.

2) Procedure

(1) Two-stage procedure

A sural nerve is harvested by perineural dissection through multiple horizontal incisions. The distal end is cut near lateral malleolus and the proximal end near 1/3 point of proximal calf. After bilateral facelift incisions were made, a zygomatic branch and a buccal branch of the facial nerve on the healthy side are identified using a nerve stimulator. The nerve endings are placed in the subcutaneous layer of the affected-side cheek. In addition, the hypoglossal nerve of the affected side is connected to the main buccal branch of the affected side after 30% partial neurotomy in a side-to-side fashion via a sural nerve interposition graft. When the Tinel's sign was observed at the grafted nerve ending after a period of time, the second stage of the operation is performed where the two sural graft endings are anastomosed with the zygomatic and main buccal branches in an end-to-end fashion (**Figure 21-16**).[11]

(2) Single stage procedure

A facelift incision is made only on the affected side and dissection is performed until the facial trunk is identified. The zygomatic, buccal, marginal mandibu-lar branches of the facial nerve and the hypoglossal nerve / masseter nerve are identified by using a nerve stimulator. The hypoglossal nerve is identified near the facial artery, 1–2 cm below the mandibular border. The masseter nerve is identified approximately 3 cm anterior to the tragus, 1 cm inferior to the zygomatic arch, and 1.5 cm deep to the SMAS (**Figure 21-17**).

A branch of the contralateral facial nerve is identified through a separate minimal incision, and subcutaneous tunneling is done in the upper lip. This incision starts from the point where a vertical line from the lateral eyebrow and the horizontal line connecting the tragus and mid-philtrum meet. It extends supero-medially for the vertical line from the lateral canthus aligned with a skin tension line 2–4 cm in length. The harvested sural nerve is passed through the tunnel and an end-to end neurorrhaphy is performed between both sides of the zygomatic branches and buccal branches via sural nerve interposition grafting (**Figure 21-18a**).

After 30% partial neurotomy, the hypoglossal nerve of the affected side is side-to-side anastomosed to a branch of the affected facial nerve via sural nerve grafting (**Figure 21-18b**).[11]

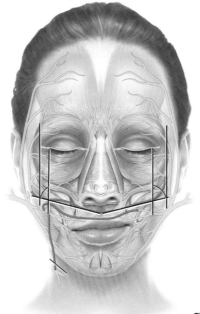
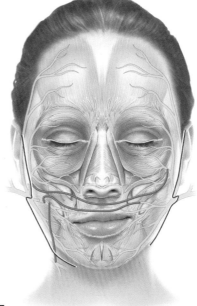

Figure 21-17.

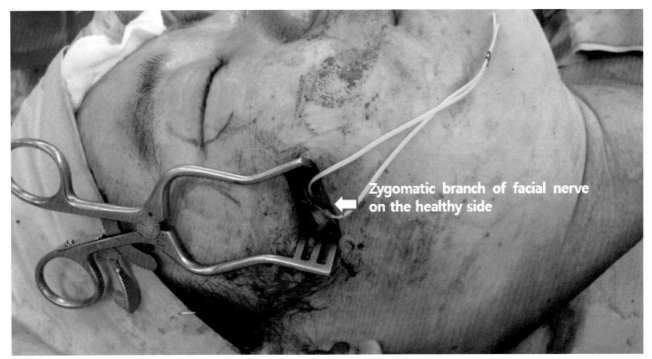

Figure 21-18a.

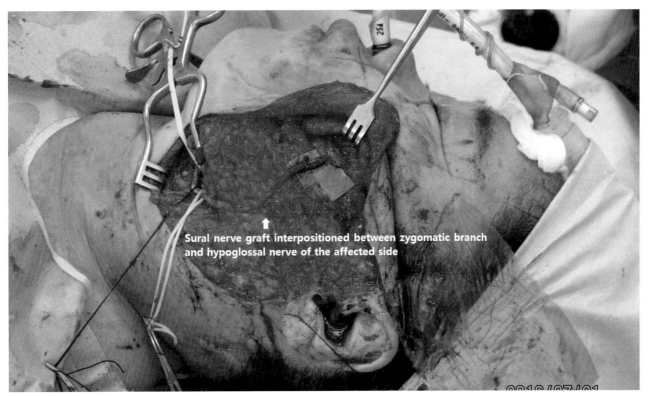

Figure 21-18b.

3) Tip and summary

The hypoglossal / masseter nerve provides not only the voluntary smile but also a fast and reliable innervation source to minimize the de-innervation atrophy of muscles until the contralateral facial nerve innervation is proceded to achieve a spontaneous smile.

2. Temporalis muscle transfer

1) Introduction

- Indication

Patients who are not suitable candidates or who have fear for free muscle transplantation may be candidates for temporalis muscle transfer.
- Pre-operative preparation or check points

The bilateral nasolabial folds should be clearly identified and marked to make sure which points to anchor the muscle and pull upward. Furthermore, which vector to pull the oral commissure should be thoroughly discussed with the patient before the operation (Figure 21-20).

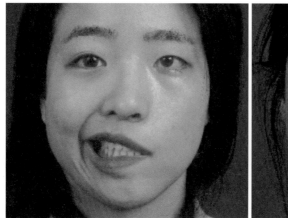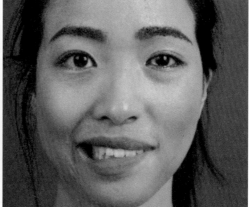

Figure 21-19. Preoperative and postoperative photographs

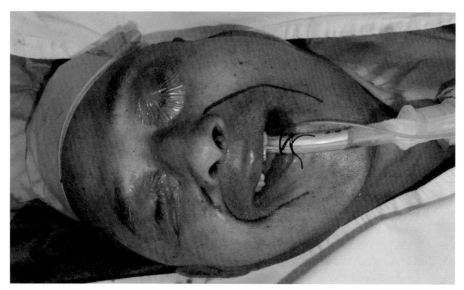

Figure 21-20.

2) Procedure

Through an intraoral gingivobuccal incision, the temporalis muscle is completely detached from its insertion at the coronoid process of mandible, and brought forward by osteomizing the tip of coronoid process. Then, another intraoral incision is made around the nasolabial fold, and submucosal tunneling is done from the first incision to the second incision.

When designing the intraoral incision lines, the Stenson's duct opening should be identified first. Also, special attention is needed to avoid injuries to the Stenson's duct when tunneling through the submucosal layer. The detached end of temporalis muscle is tunneled through the buccal fat pad and is fixated along the nasolabial fold and oral commissure usually at 4-5 points with non-absorbable sutures (**Figure 21-21a, 21b**).[12]

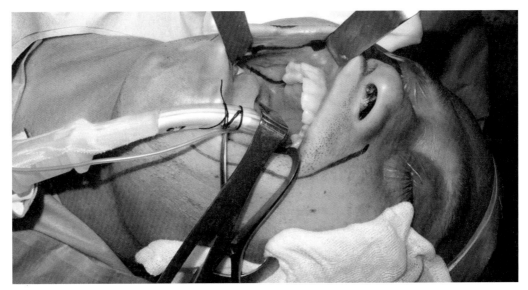

Figure 21-21a.

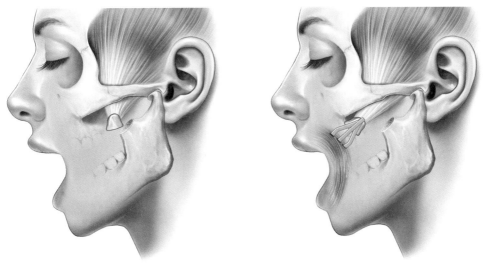

Figure 21-21b.

3) Tip and Summary

Overcorrection of the oral commissure is needed because the amount of lift loosens a certain amount as time passes.

This technique has a great advantage of avoiding dissection at the origin of the temporalis muscle, thus simplifying the procedure with less scars and ensuring an enhanced blood supply.

3. Free partial Latissimus dorsi transfer

1) Introduction

- Indication

Patients with ability to undergo a substantial operative procedure with general anesthesia and who accept the morbidity of the donor sites can be candidates of this procedure. Because older patients have a risk of failure of reinnervation, young patients are generally more recommended.

- Pre-operative preparation or check points

Careful analysis of the patient's smile on the non-paralyzed side is required to establish a symmetric smile. It is important to assess the direction of movement of the oral commissure and upper lip.

2) Procedure

A partial LD muscle flap is elevated including the thoracodorsal artery and vein as the vascular pedicles and the descending branch of thoracodorsal nerve as the innervation source. The transverse branch is preserved by splitting the proximal portion of thoracodorsal nerve interfascicularly and confirming the intactness of the nerve with a nerve stimulator (**Figure 21-23a, 23b, 23c**).[13,14]

The harvested flap is inset in the paralyzed side of the face with the vascular pedicles anastomosed to either the facial artery/ vein or the superficial temporal artery/ vein. The proximal end of the thoracodorsal nerve is coaptated with the contralateral buccal branch and the distal portion of descending branch with the ipsilateral masseter nerve (**Figure 21-23d**).[15]

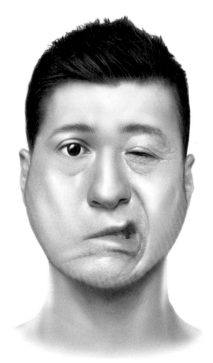
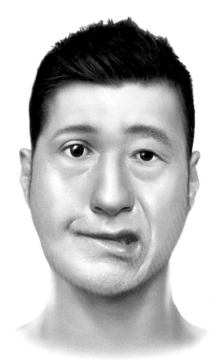

Figure 21-22. Preoperative and postoperative photographs

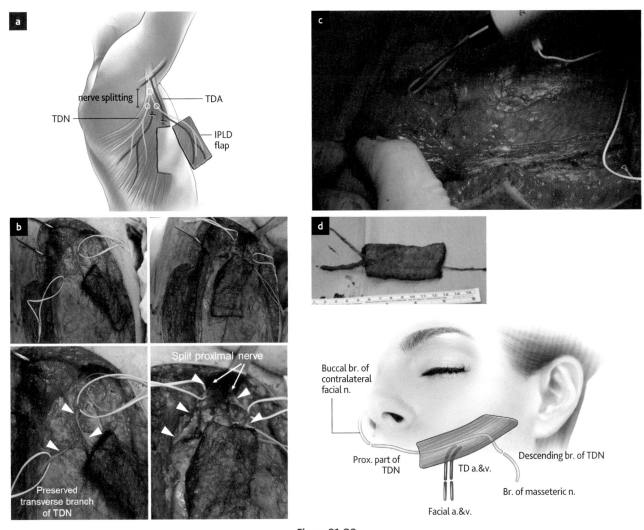

Figure 21-23.

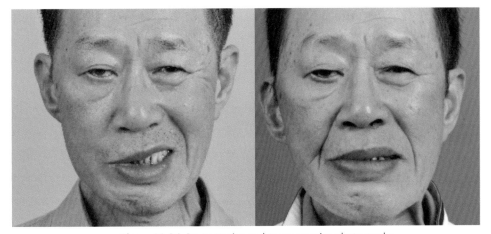

Figure 21-24. Preoperative and postoperative photographs

VI. Tip and summary

This method involves a retrograde innervation of the descending branch of thoracodorsal nerve. Although there is not much evidence reported on the efficacy of retrograde innervation in facial nerve reconstruction, there have been several animal studies that suggested the comparability of reverse-oriented nerve regeneration.[16-17] In our experience, there was no significant difference between the retrograde and antegrade innervation of transplanted muscle flap.

REFERENCES

1. Freilinger G, Gruber H, Happak W, Pechmann U. Surgical anatomy of the mimic muscle system and the facial nerve: importance for reconstructive and aesthetic surgery. Plast Reconstr Surg 1987;80(5):686-90.

2. Davis RA, Anson BJ, Budinger JM, Kurth LR. Surgical anatomy of the facial nerve and parotid gland based upon a study of 350 cervicofacial halves. Surg Gynecol Obstet 1956;102(4):385-412.

3. Ishikawa Y. An anatomical study on the distribution of the temporal branch of the facial nerve. J Craniomaxillofac Surg 1990;18(7):287-92.

4. Westin LM, Zuker R. A new classification system for facial paralysis in the clinical setting. J Craniofac Surg 2003;14(5):672-9.

5. Manktelow RT. Use of the gold weight for lagophthalmos. Oper tech plast reconstr surg 1999;6(3):157-8.

6. Hayashi A, Yoshizawa H, Natori Y, Senda D, Tanaka R, Mizuno H. Levator lengthening technique using cartilage or fascia graft for paralytic lagophthalmos in facial paralysis. J Plast Reconstr Aesthet Surg 2016;69(5):679-86.

7. Park HJ, Chang H. Static treatment of incomplete facial paralysis with tensor fascia lata sling. J Korean Skull Base Soc 2019;14(2):39-43.

8. Yoleri L, Songur E, Mavioglu H, et al. Cross-facial nerve grafting as an adjunct to hyperglossal-facial nerve crossover in reanimation of early facial paralysis: clinical and electrophysiological evaluation. Ann Plast Surg 2001;46:301-7.

9. Braam MJ, Nicolai JP. Axonal regeneration rate through cross-face nerve grafts. Microsurgery 1993;14:589-91.

10. Klebuc MJ. Facial reanimation using the masseter to facial nerve transfer. Plast Reconstr Surg 2011;127(5):1909-15.

11. Park SO, Ha JH, Kim IK, Jin US, Chang H. Single-stage cross-facial nerve grafting has a result equivalent to that of two-stage cross-facial nerve grafting. Microsurgery 2020 Feb;40(2):175-82.

12. Park DJ, Chung JH, Baek SO, Kim JW, Hwang NH, Yoon ES, Lee BI, Park SH. Intraoral temporalis transposition for facial reanimation: A novel technique in facial nerve palsy. J Craniomaxillofac Surg 2020 Mar;48(3):235-41.

13. Kwon ST, Chang H, Oh M. Anatomic basis of interfascicular nerve splitting of innervated partial latissimus dorsi muscle flap. J Plast Reconstr Aesthet Surg 2011 May;64(5):e109-14.

14. Park SO, Kim J, Kim IK, Chung JH, Jin US, Chang H. Minimizing donor site morbidity using the interfascicular nerve splitting technique in single-stage latissimus neuromuscular transfer for facial reanimation. J Plast Reconstr Aesthet Surg 2020 Nov 5:S1748-6815(20)30526-X.

15. Manktelow RT, Tomat LR, Zuker RM, et al. Smile reconstruction in adults with free muscle transfer innervated by the masseter motor nerve: effectiveness and cerebral adaptation. Plast Reconstr Surg 2006;118:885-899.

16. Nakatsuka H, Takamatsu K, Koshimune M, Imai Y, Enomoto M, Yamano Y. Experimental study of polarity in reversing cable nerve grafts. J Reconstr Microsurg 2002 Aug;18(6):509-15.

17. Kurita M, Yamazaki K, Eto H, Seike S, Takushima A, Harii K. Reinnervation of segmented latissimus dorsi muscle with the distal stump of the thoracodorsal nerve: A preliminary experimental study in rats. Microsurgery 2013 Oct;33(7):545-50.

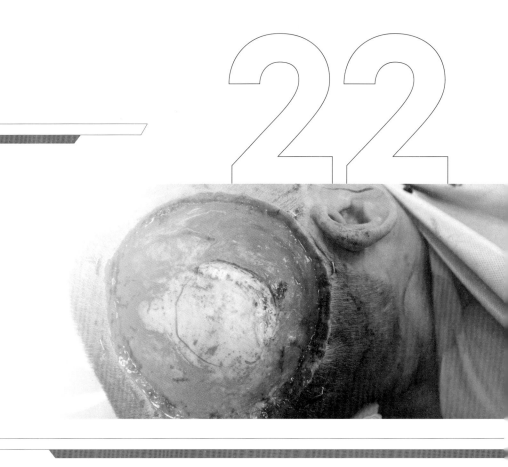

22

SCALP
RECONSTRUCTION

Jong Won Hong M.D., Ph.D.

I. Introduction

The scalp is a thin, yet highly vascular, structure that covers the entire skull. From the perspective of reconstructive surgeons, the scalp is a good flap because of its abundant blood flow, but it is limited by a lack of redundant tissue. For these reasons, wound healing itself is usually good, but paradoxically, it can be difficult to repair a soft tissue defect with the remaining nearby tissue.

The biologic activity of the scalp is high, contributing to the need for an abundant blood supply. Much of this activity involves the constant growth of hair. The scalp is also an area of pronounced sweating (e.g., during exercise) and release of much body heat.

The scalp consists of 5 main layers: the skin, dense connective tissue (subcutaneous fat), aponeurosis (aponeurotic layer), loose connective tissue, and periosteum (pericranium) (**Figure 22-1**). Few textbooks explain these layers in detail. The outer layer of the bony skull (periosteum) is covered by a layer of loose connective tissue, which is usually known as the galea. However, several references describe the aponeurosis and loose connective tissue as the galea aponeurotica and loose areolar tissue, respectively. Thus, the term "galea" is sometimes used to refer to the area between the dense connective tissue and periosteum, containing both the aponeurotic and the loose connective tissue layers.

When we perform blunt dissection, it is usually quite easy to determine when the aponeurosis (aponeurotic layer) deep to the dense connective tissue has been reached, as the aponeurosis is relatively avascular and often feels like a "space" over the galea and periosteum. The galea may or may not be firmly attached to the periosteum. If we scrape the base of the scalp by applying direct force, the galea can be detached from the periosteum, allowing elevation of a scalp flap including the galea. However, if we dissect over the aponeurosis without directly scraping the base of the scalp, the galea will remain with the periosteum, and the flap will not include the galea. Thus, when we

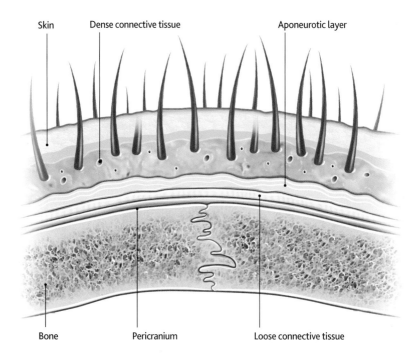

Skin — Dense connective tissue — Aponeurotic layer

Bone — Pericranium — Loose connective tissue

Figure 22-1. Five layers of the scalp: the skin, dense connective tissue, aponeurosis, loose connective tissue, and periosteum. The aponeurosis (aponeurotic layer) is a relatively avascular plane. Most of the scalp vessel network is located in the dense connective tissue layer.

elevate a "scalp" flap, the skin and dense connective tissue are lifted together as essentially one mass, and if we dissect loosely in the aponeurotic "space", we can elevate a scalp flap leaving the loose connective (areolar) tissue and periosteum in place. The aponeurosis will or will not be included in the scalp flap, depending on the dissection scraping force. If we dissect down to the periosteum and elevate deep to the periosteum,

we can obtain a scalp flap including the periosteum as well. When the goal is to use a galeal flap, it is better to elevate the scalp via or over the aponeurotic "space" without forceful scraping, leaving the galea on the base of the scalp. Galeal flap elevation is easier to perform from the base than from an elevated scalp (**Figure 22-2**).

Scalp blood flow from the forehead to the parietal

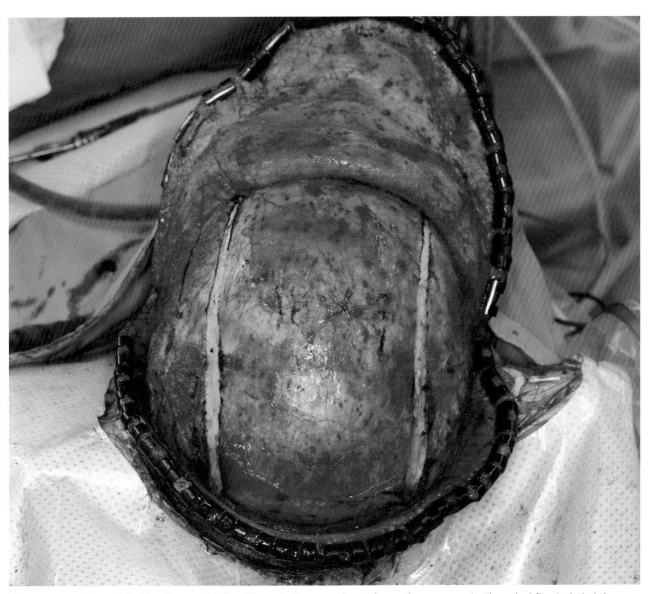

Figure 22-2. Design and incision for a galeal flap. The scalp flap was elevated over the aponeurosis. The galeal flap included the aponeurosis and loose connective tissue. The main superficial temporal vessels are usually included in scalp flaps, as they are located in the dense connective tissue layer.

bones is supplied mainly by the superficial temporal artery and vein. These vessels also cover some occipital areas. The occipital area is additionally supplied by the occipital artery and vein. These vessels are quite large, with abundant blood flow, and are all sufficient for large flap recipient vessels.

Where is the main superficial temporal vessel network when a scalp flap is elevated? It is located in the dense connective tissue layer. Therefore, the superficial temporal artery and vein are usually present in a scalp flap, so if we elevate a scalp flap over the aponeurosis, these vessels will not remain on the base of the scalp. When using the superficial temporal vessels, we must be careful to not apply traction when flipping over the scalp, especially with bicoronal incisions.

There are several issues with scalp defects. First, limited tissue exists around these defects, so primary repair can be surprisingly difficult, even with small defects. Second, the presence of a bone defect, previous radiotherapy, or infection will make the remaining tissue more difficult to use. Third, several reasons for scalp defects originate from within the cranium. Even if the scalp itself is healthy, repeated infections or chronic wounds may arise from intracranial pathology, which must be resolved simultaneously. Fourth, the forehead is a particularly significant region, as it important from an aesthetic perspective, and the facial nerve passes through the area. Fifth, scalp hair is also important for a cosmetic point. Patients are often more worried about hair damage and scalp scars than other scalp problems.

II. Procedures

There are 5 main reconstruction methods for scalp defects: primary repair, local flap advancement, local flap transposition and skin graft, tissue expander, and free flap.

1. Primary repair

Primary repair is performed in a standard manner, but it is important to distribute the scalp tension evenly during subcutaneous suturing. Forces applied to the

subcutaneous sutures should only be used for making knots. If force is also used to pull tissue, the tissue may be damaged or the suture may break. If the scalp is pulled with nylon suture to adjust the approximation, scalp tissue can be easily injured, leading to wound dehiscence and secondary infection because of necrosis of the scalp margin. Even if the condition of the scalp tissue improves later, secondary bone or intracranial infection may cause continuing wound problems (**Figure 22-3**). When significant tension is present, it is useful to temporarily align the defect edges using a towel clip or stapler during subcutaneous suturing.

2. Local flap advancement

Even if the defect is small, limited amount of redundant scalp tissue exists after adolescence; this can be overcome with undermining scalp dissection. This undermining is performed in the aponeurotic "space" over the loose connective tissue. When dissection occurs deep to the periosteum, the periosteum is not redundant and does not elongate. If the extent of dissection is wide, it is difficult to control bleeding in the deeper areas; therefore, careful dissection is important (**Figure 22-4**).

3. Local flap transposition and skin graft

If wide dissection is difficult or flap advancement and repair is difficult, a partial tension-release additional incision can be performed. Thus, the original defect would be covered with a scalp flap, and the new healthy defect created for tension release would be covered with a skin graft.

The flap can be designed as a lobed flap, but rotation may not work well. Blood flow originates from one side in a lobed flap, and the proximal part of this flap is easily overlapped or crumpled during the rotation. If this part is cut, the width on the side of the blood flow will be narrower. A bipedicled flap is another, often better, option. This flap receives blood flow from both sides and is easy to move. There is also no overlapping part after insetting the flap.

With regard to the newly created defect site, a skin graft is possible only when the galea or periosteum remains at the site (**Figure 22-5**).

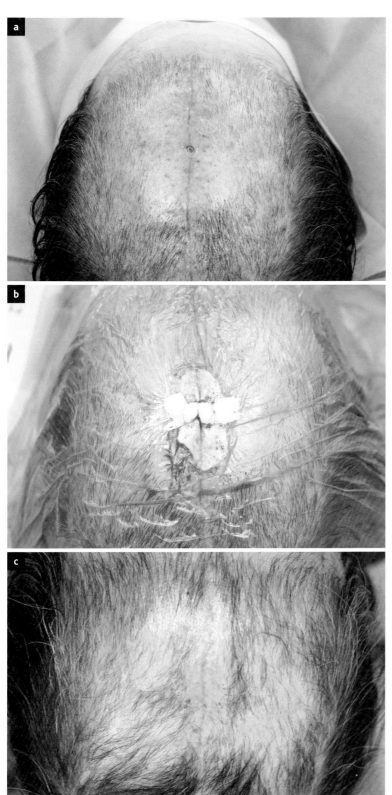

Figure 22-3. Focal scalp defect. Although the scalp defect is small, limited tissue is available to cover the defect. If the cause of the defect is a chronic wound, it is especially difficult to repair. (a) Focal defect in a chronic wound. (b) The remaining scalp in the area was thin, requiring the use of a pillow suture instead of a subcutaneous suture. (c) Defect at 2 months after surgery.

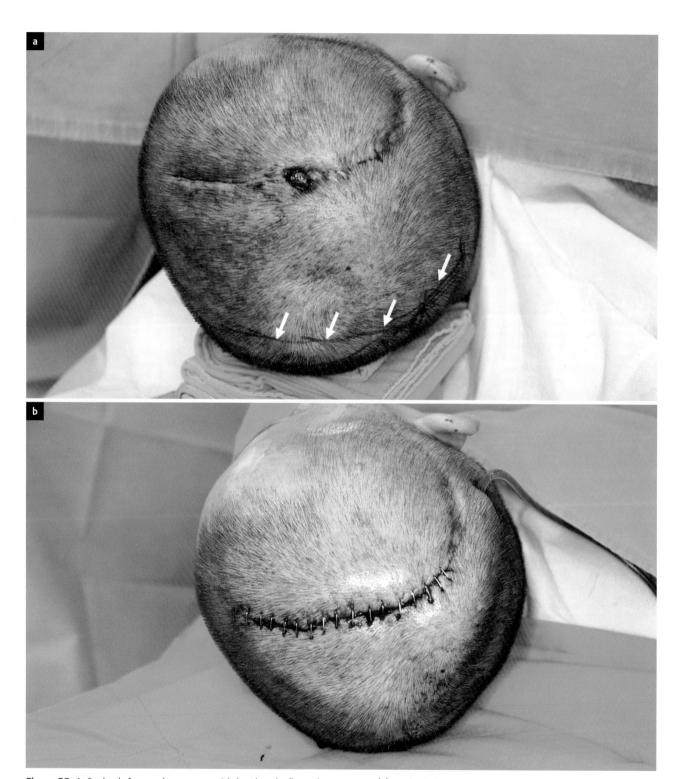

Figure 22-4. Scalp defect and coverage with local scalp flap advancement. (a) Scalp defect at an incision and osteotome site resulting from a chronic wound. Scalp flap dissection and undermining in a large area were extended to the proximal part of the right temporalis and to the left temporalis over the parietal area. Bipedicled flap transposition was considered as an alternative ("plan B"), as indicated by the additional incision line (white arrows) drawn for this plan. (b) Repair was successfully performed via huge scalp flap advancement.

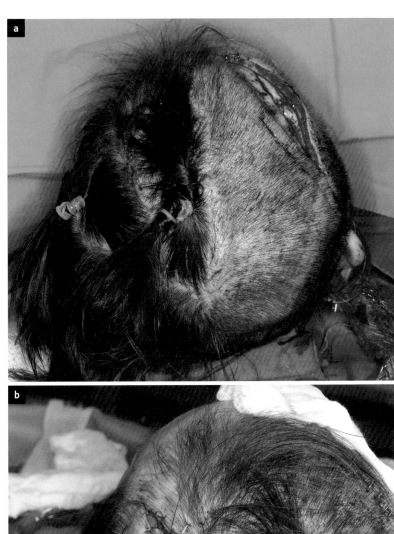

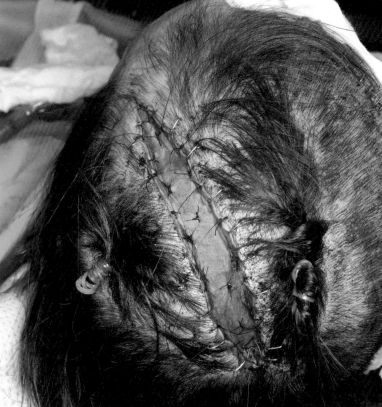

Figure 22-5. Scalp defect and coverage with a bilobed flap and skin graft. (a) Original scalp defect with exposed bone. (b) A releasing incision was performed on the opposite site. Undermining must be done over the periosteum or loose connective tissue. A skin graft was inserted at the "new" scalp defect.

4. Tissue expander

A tissue expander is very useful for scalp reconstruction. It is a unique reconstruction method that allows the defect to be covered with hair. Even during the expansion phase, the area does not appear completely empty. However, use of an expander requires 3 steps, instead of 1-stage reconstruction: tissue expander insertion, expansion, and coverage with an expanded flap.

When selecting tissue expanders, the type and number are determined by comprehensively considering the defect size and the location where the tissue expander(s) will be placed. The projection (final height) is an especially important determinant of the extent of advancement of the expanded flap. Although the base may be wide, the moving distance will be quite short if the height is low.

There are various tissue expander shapes that can be used, depending on the shape and location of the defect, but it is best to have the largest surface area in full expansion. Thus, a rectangular expander is usually the best shape. If a too-large tissue expander is located on the side of the head (i.e., in the temple or occipital regions), it may gradually move downward during ex-

pansion because of its weight. To avoid this, multiple smaller expanders could be used instead (**Figure 22-6**).

5. Free flap

When a free flap is chosen, the most important consideration is to clearly secure the pedicle. The superficial temporal vessels are generally used as recipient vessels, but these vessels should be assessed by direct vision intraoperatively after vessel dissection. Occasionally, the superficial temporal vein is too small or variable, although the superficial temporal artery is adequate. In this situation, the facial artery or vein is used. This results in a significantly longer donor vessel. If the pedicle is not long enough, the flap itself may require lowering to the bottom of the face by designing a larger flap.

After recipient vessels are dissected, they should not be cut until the vessel anastomoses are performed. The status of the vessels can be checked by assessing pulsations and by gently wiggling the vessels. Scalp vessels are more tortuous than other vessels and are prone to spasm. It is therefore better to maintain vessel patency before anastomosis (**Figure 22-7**).

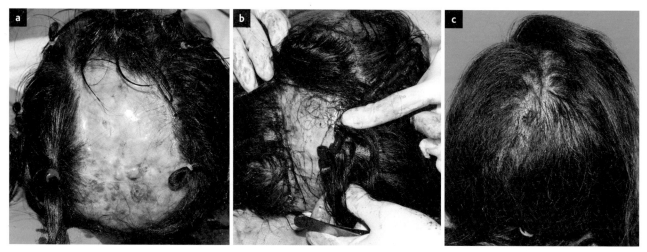

Figure 22-6. Scalp reconstruction using a tissue expander. (a) Tissue expander insertion is the first step. Surgeon must choose the tissue expander by considering the defect and the status of the healthy scalp. (b) Reconstruction using an expanded flap. Several tissue expanders and serial expansions were used for this patient. (c) Final result of the reconstruction.

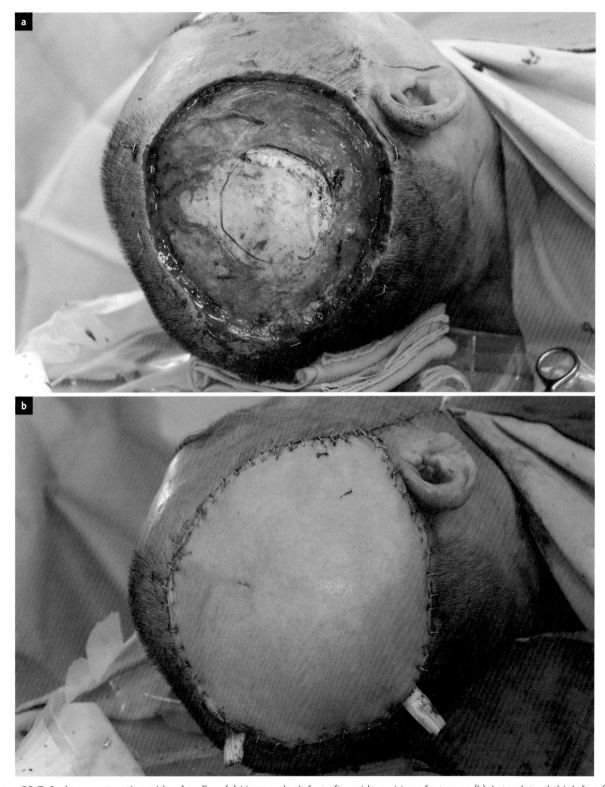

Figure 22-7. Scalp reconstruction with a free flap. (a) Huge scalp defect after wide excision of a tumor. (b) Anterolateral thigh free flap used for reconstruction.

III. Tips and summary

1. It is necessary to understand not only the characteristics of the scalp but also the status of the bone and underlying intracranium.

2. The cause of the scalp defect must be identified. The reconstruction surgeon should also carefully review the previous surgical records, the reason for the surgery, whether the area received radiotherapy, the condition of the skull bone, and the condition of the underlying intracranial area. If the cause of the defect is skull osteoporosis or infection of an artificial dura mater, there is a high possibility of recurrence, even after the scalp defect is closed. In addition, the reconstruction surgeon should check the plans for management after scalp reconstruction to determine whether subsequent plans will disturb the reconstruction or whether the reconstruction will disturb subsequent management plans.

3. The method of reconstruction must be decided by considering the patient's status. Reconstruction surgeons must establish a "plan B" to be used if the original approach fails. This is particularly important for scalp defects because of the limited amount of redundant tissue.

4. Prevention is best. To reduce the likelihood of postoperative scalp defects, it is recommended that the incision line and skull osteotome line not coincide. This will prevent the osteotome edge from irritating the incision wound, and if there is an incision wound problem, it will not extend to the bone and intracranium.

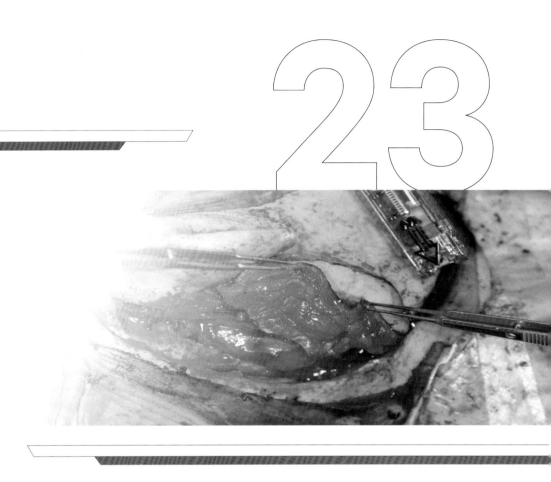

23

USEFUL FLAPS FOR SKULL BASE RECONSTRUCTIONS

Ho Jin Park M.D., Ph.D., Tae Suk Oh M.D., Ph.D.,
Jong Woo Choi M.D., Ph.D.

I. Introduction

Skull base neoplasm is one of the challenging tumors to manage. The complex anatomy of the skull base makes resection difficult. Because of the proximity of the dura to the paranasal sinuses and nasopharynx following tumor resection, the skull base surgery increases the risk for complication and morbidity after tumor resection. Cerebrospinal fluid leak, meningitis, and osteomyelitis are relatively common major complications after skull base surgery.[1] In the past, skull base surgeries were accompanied by major complications due to limited reconstructive options. However, with the recent advances in microsurgical techniques, free tissue transfer enables surgeons to reconstruct complex defects with minimizing such major complications. Free tissue transfer has become the mainstay of skull base reconstruction.

Irish et al. divided the skull base into three zones, and different reconstructive options were applied for each zone. An anatomical structure bounds each zone[2] (**Figure 23-1**). Zone I is bounded from the anterior midline to the posterior wall of the orbit and includes an extension to the foramen magnum. Zone II involves the infratemporal and pterygomaxillary fossae and the overlying segment of the middle cranial fossa. It ranges from the posterior wall of the orbit to the posterior aspect of the petrous temporal bone. Lastly, zone III includes the posterior cranial fossa and posterior segment of the middle cranial fossa.

In this chapter, the author reviews the reconstruction methods of skull base defects according to the zone.

II. Procedures

1. Zone I reconstruction

Zone I tumors generally arise from the sinuses, orbit, and midfacial skin and may invade the cribriform plate and dura. The reconstruction method is determined by the size, location, and required tissue type. If there is a defect in the dura, tensor fascia lata grafts are used to repair it. Various type of local flaps, including glabella flap and forehead flap, has been introduced for small zone 1 defect. The pericarnial flap can be used for sinusoidal lining or soft tissue coverage in a small zone I defect with low donor site morbidity.[3,4] In case of a more lateral skull base defect, a temporal muscle flap can be employed. However, it cannot be used if the vascular pedicle of the temporalis is damaged during tumor resection, and temporal depression deformity may occur following muscle transposition.

Free tissue transfer is the best reconstructive option in the medium to large zone I defect.[5,6] Free tissue transfer can provide well vascularized and bulky tissue. Unlike the regional flap, the free tissue transfer is not limited by pedicle length and is easy to inset the flap at the desired position. Thin fasciocutaneous flaps, such as radial forearm flap and anterolateral thigh flap, are commonly used to zone I defect because they well contour the skull shape. If the defect is large and bulky tissue is required, a rectus abdominis myocutaneous flap may be used.

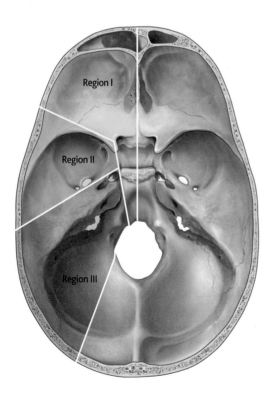

Figure 23-1. Skull base regions

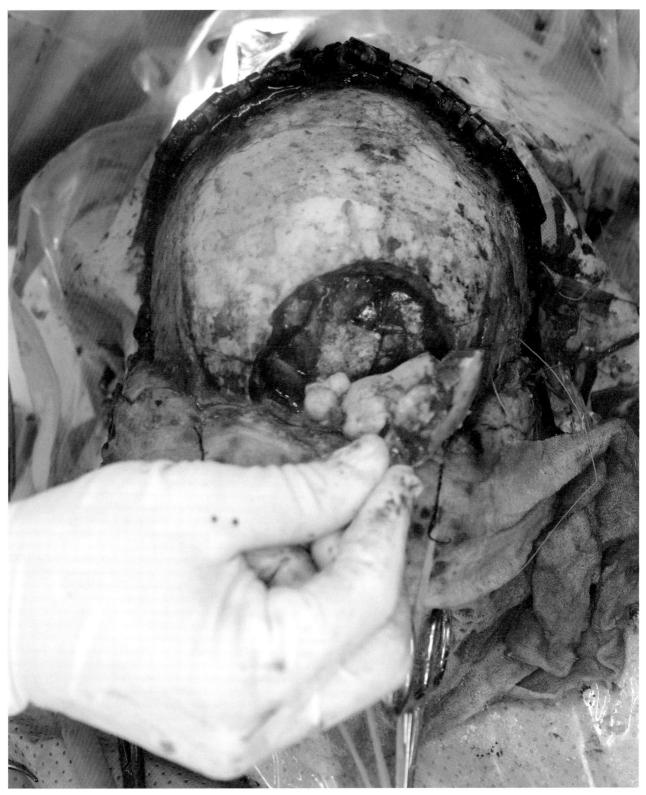

Figure 23-2. Zone I defect. After resection of osteoma on the frontal area, the patient had anterior cranial fossa and frontal bone defect.

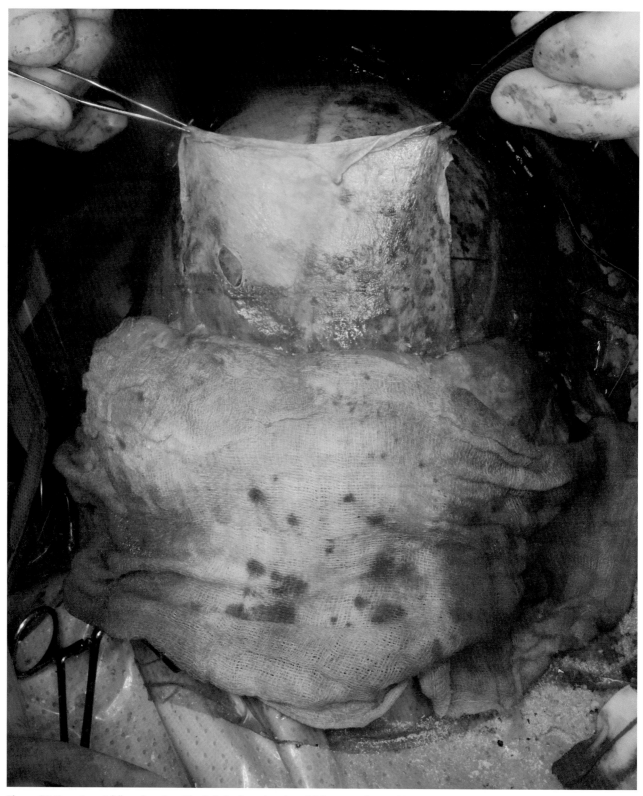

Figure 23-3. pericranial flap elevation. The inferior-based pericranial flap was elevated from the calvarium.

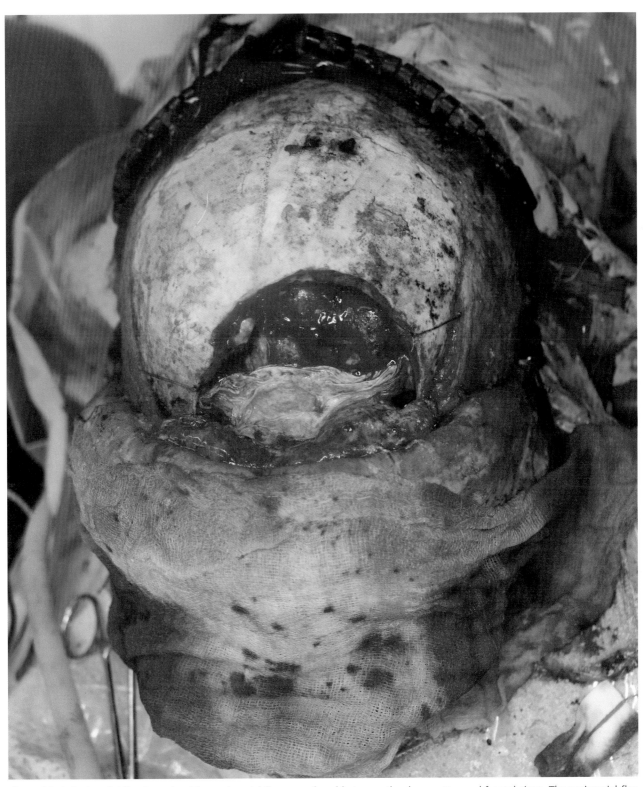

Figure 23-4. Pericranial flap insetting. The pericranial flap was placed between the dura matter and frontal sinus. The pericranial flap acted as a barrier between the nasal cavity and the anterior cranial fossa.

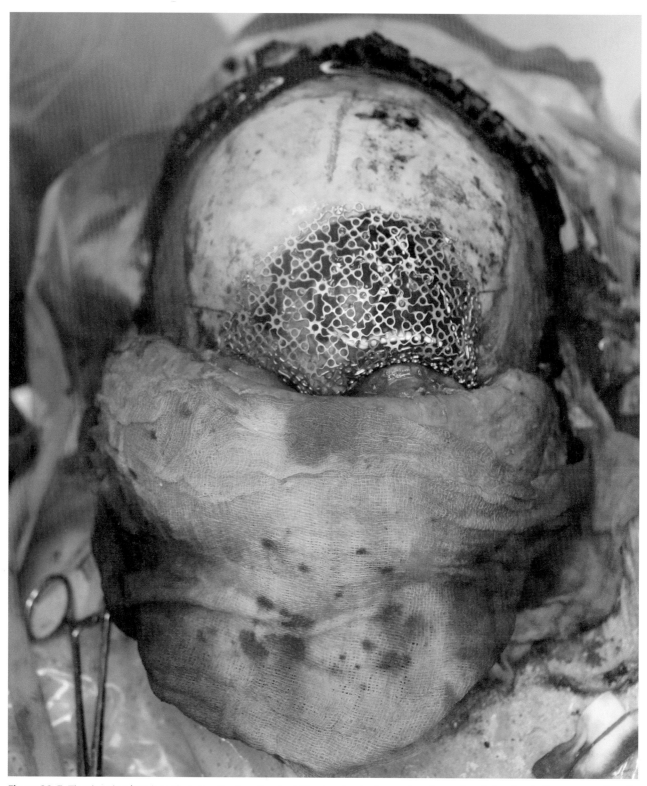

Figure 23-5. Titanium implant insertion. A patient-customized titanium implant was placed over the defect for skull reconstruction. By implanting the titanium implant, forehead depression can be avoided.

2. Zone II reconstruction

Zone II neoplasm is originated from nasopharyngeal cancer, clival chordoma, meningiomas, and invasion of ear, scalp, or parotid neoplasm.[2] Several major vascular and neural structures are included in zone II. The internal carotid artery, maxillary and mandibular branches of the trigeminal nerve, facial nerve, and auditory nerves traverse this zone. Therefore, zone II defects can be accompanied by these major structural defects.

For facial nerve defect reconstruction, the sural nerve can be interposed between the facial nerve trunk and facial nerve branches.[7] The methods of soft tissue coverage are determined by the defect size. Small defects located laterally may be covered using a temporalis muscle flap. Historically, regional flaps, such as pectoralis major flap and trapezius flap had been used, but free tissue transfer is more advocated these days.[8] Since the zone II defects may include maxillary cavity or mastoid process, dead space obliteration is required. Bulky free flaps like anterolateral thigh flap and rectus abdominis myocutaneous flap are often used for soft tissue coverage and dead space obliteration.

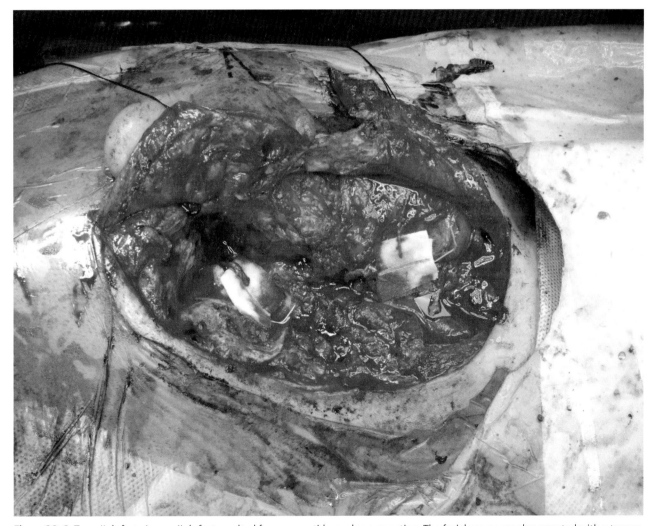

Figure 23-6. Zone II defect. A zone II defect resulted from a parotid neoplasm resection. The facial nerve was also resected with a tumor.

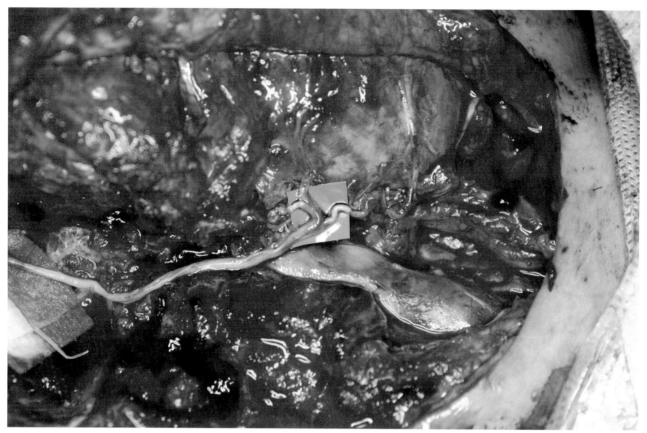

Figure 23-7. Sural nerve graft. The sural nerve was grafted from the facial nerve trunk to the zygomatic and buccal branches of the facial nerve.

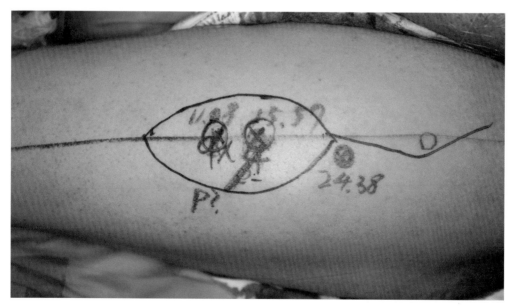

Figure 23-8. Anterolateral thigh flap harvest. The 9×4 cm sized anterolateral flap was designed on the patients' left leg.

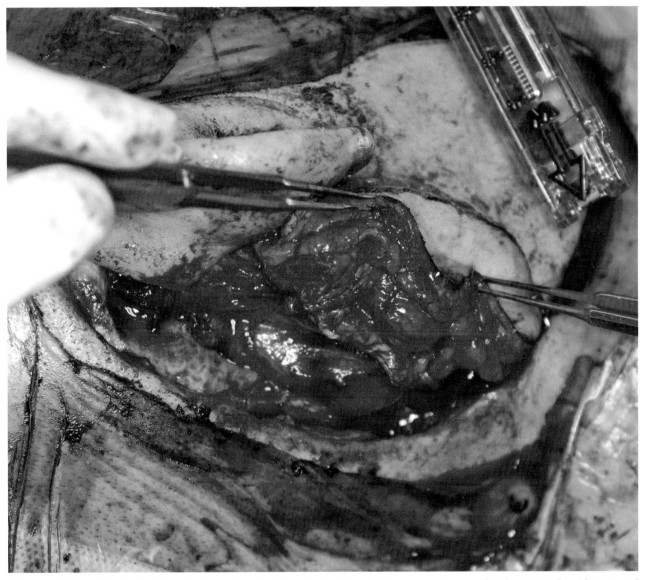

Figure 23-9. Anterolateral thigh flap insetting. The anterolateral thigh flap pedicles were anastomosed with superior thyroid artery and external jugular vein. Then, the flap covered the defect area.

3. Zone III reconstruction

Neural and vascular structures like internal jugular vein, glossopharyngeal nerve, hypoglossal nerve, vagus nerve and accessory nerve included in the zone III. Zone III defects may involve these neural and vascular structures. The common tumors in Zone III are glomus tumor, schwannoma and squamous cell carcinoma.[9] As in zone II reconstruction, the free tissue transfer is primary choice of reconstruction in zone III defect. The anterolateral thigh and rectus abdominis myocutaneous free flaps are emoplyed in this region when a larger flap is needed.[10]

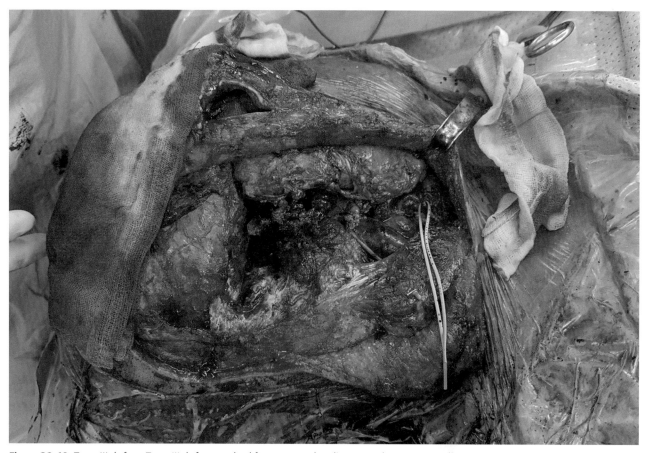

Figure 23-10. Zone III defect. Zone III defect resulted from external auditory canal squamous cell carcinoma resection.

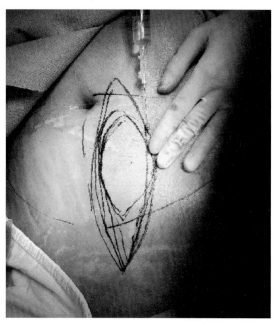

Figure 23-11. Vertical rectus abdominis flap harvest. A vertical rectus abdominis (VRAM) flap was selected because the defect size was extensive, and a large volume of the flap was required to obliterate dead space. The flap was designed based on the inferior epigastric vascular pedicle.

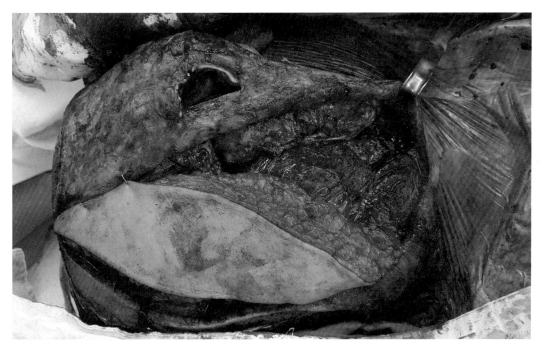

Figure 23-12. Vascular anastomosis. The VRAM flap pedicels were anastomosed with superficial temporal artery and internal jugular vein branch.

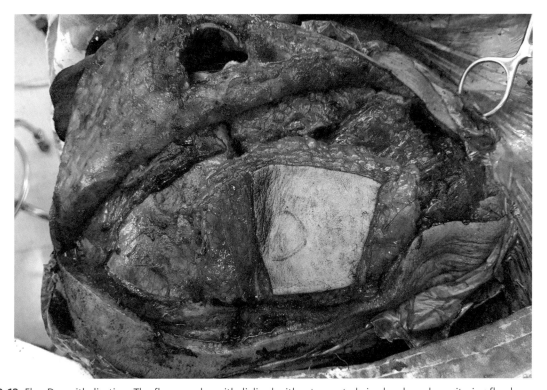

Figure 23-13. Flap De-epithelization. The flap was de-epithelialized without a central circular-shaped monitoring flap because the skin defect was minor in this case.

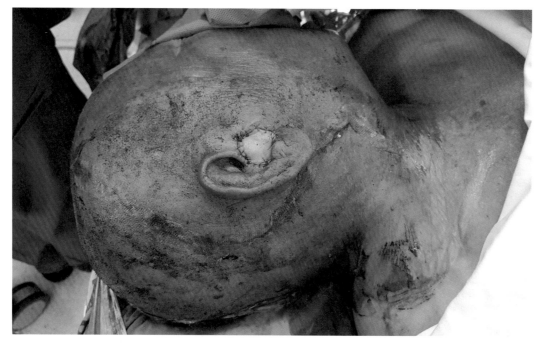

Figure 23-14. The VRAM flap inset. The VRAM flap was placed under the skin flap and a monitoring flap was located around the external auditory canal.

III. Tip & Summary

1. The skull base is a complex area to reconstruct because of its location, the numerous vital structures, and the unique function of the various anatomic structures.

2. Free tissue transfer is the preferred method in skull base defect when the defect is extensive, and a significant area of soft tissue coverage is necessary. Well-vascularized tissue provides an excellent dural seal and protection from infection sources.

3. Local flaps, such as pericranial flap and temporalis flap, can be used in small defects. The local flap is available when the defect is in proximity with the flap, and the flap vascularity is preserved.

4. The water-tight dural seal is important to protect intracranial contents from the nasal cavity and potential infection sources.

5. Sinuses, cavities, and dead spaces must be obliterated to prevent seroma and subsequent infection.

REFERENCES

1. Gullane PJ, Lipa JE, Novak CB, Neligan PC. Reconstruction of skull base defects. Clin Plast Surg 2005;32:391-39, vii.

2. Irish JC, Gullane PJ, Gentili F, et al. Tumors of the skull base: outcome and survival analysis of 77 cases. Head Neck 1994;16:3-10.

3. Noone MC, Osguthorpe JD, Patel S. Pericranial flap for closure of paramedian anterior skull base defects. Otolaryngol Head Neck Surg 2002;127:494-500.

4. Chang DW, Langstein HN, Gupta A, et al. Reconstructive management of cranial base defects after tumor ablation. Plast Reconstr Surg 2001;107:1346-1355; discussion 1356-47.

5. Califano J, Cordeiro PG, Disa JJ, et al. Anterior cranial base reconstruction using free tissue transfer: changing trends. Head Neck 2003;25:89-96.

6. Neligan PC, Mulholland S, Irish J, et al. Flap selection in cranial base reconstruction. Plast Reconstr Surg 1996;98:1159-1166; discussion 1167-58.

7. Gidley PW, Herrera SJ, Hanasono MM, et al. The impact of radiotherapy on facial nerve repair. Laryngoscope 2010;120:1985-89.

8. Bakamjian VY, Long M, Rigg B. Experience with the medially based deltopectoral flap in reconstructve surgery of the head and neck. Br J Plast Surg 1971;24:174-83.

9. Jones NF, Schramm VL, Sekhar LN. Reconstruction of the cranial base following tumour resection. Br J Plast Surg 1987;40:155-62.

10. Rosenthal EL, King T, McGrew BM, Carroll W, Magnuson JS, Wax MK. Evolution of a paradigm for free tissue transfer reconstruction of lateral temporal bone defects. Head Neck 2008;30:589-94.

INDEX